THE
AUTOIMMUNE
PALEO
COOKBOOK AND
ACTION PLAN

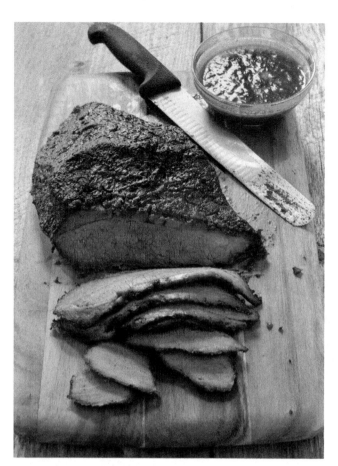

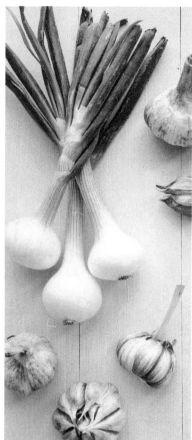

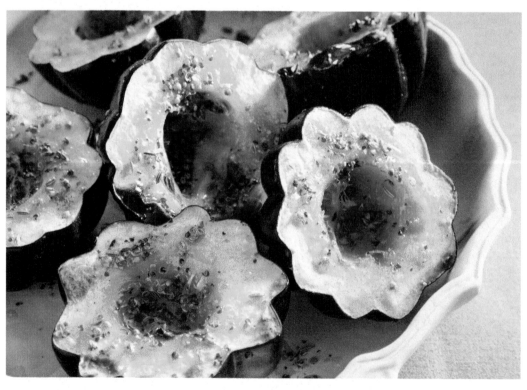

THE AUTOIMMUNE PALEO
COOKBOOK AND ACTION PLAN

A PRACTICAL GUIDE TO EASING
YOUR AUTOIMMUNE DISEASE SYMPTOMS
WITH NOURISHING FOOD

ROCKRIDGE
PRESS

Photo credits: Keller & Keller Photography/Stockfood, p. 2, top left; Danny Lerner/Stockfood, p. 2, bottom; Ina Peters/Stocksy, p. 6; Rob Fiocca Photography/Stockfood, p. 10; Pavel Gramatikov/Stocksy, p.15; Samantha Linsell/Stockfood, p. 67; Sara Remington/Stocksy, p. 68; Ina Peters/Stocksy, p. 97; Anthony Lanneretonne/Stockfood, p. 100; Rua Castilho/Stockfood, p. 132; Christina Soong-Kroeger/Stockfood, p. 164; Keller & Keller Photography/Stockfood, p. 188; Ira Leoni/Stockfood, p. 205; Sara Remington/Stocksy, p. 236; Zabert Sandmann Verlag/Jan-Peter Westermann/Stockfood, p. 254; Ina Peters/Stocksy, p. 270. All other photos www.shutterstock.com.

ISBN: Print 978-1-62315-461-5 | eBook 978-1-62315-522-3

FIVE TIPS
TO TREAT AUTOIMMUNE DISEASES THROUGH DIET

You are not destined to live your life in pain. *Autoimmune Paleo Cookbook* has valuable information about how to transform your health by using diet to heal your body. Here are some quick tips to get started on your path to wellness.

1 **Eat seasonally.** Not only are seasonal fruits and vegetables tastier, but they also are less expensive and more nutritious than foods that are not in season.

2 **Consider your gray-area foods.** Your food sensitivities and tolerances are unique to you. If you find yourself reacting to the gray-area food list, you can always eliminate these foods and try reintroducing them, one by one, when your elimination phase is over.

3 **Supplements or not?** You might already be taking supplements to manage your autoimmune disease. If they are working, don't stop.

4 **Healthy can be expensive—but there are ways around that.** Become friends with local farmers, visit farmers' markets, learn about batch cooking, and understand the value of prioritizing your food choices to get the most out of a dollar.

5 **Keep track of all your changes.** Keeping a journal or a simple notebook outlining the physical and emotional changes that occur during the course of your disease is extremely valuable.

CONTENTS

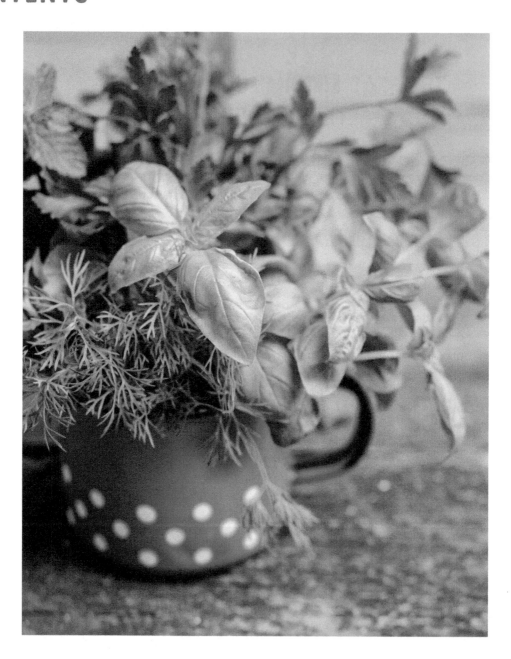

INTRODUCTION

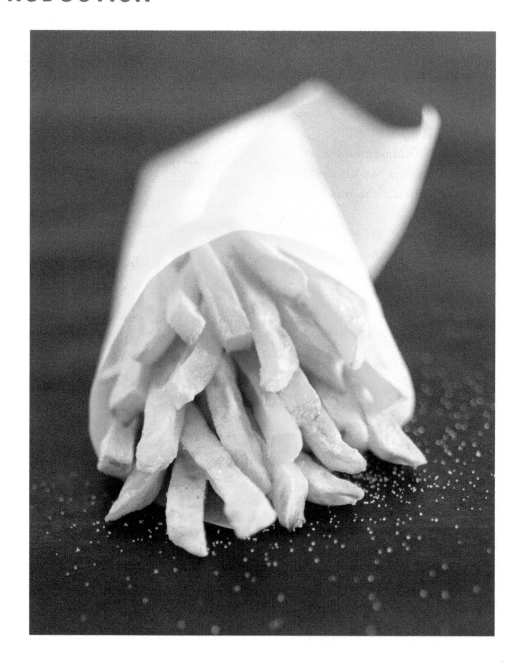

The prevalence of autoimmune diseases has skyrocketed in the past few decades. The American Autoimmune Related Diseases Association (AARDA) estimates that approximately 50 million people in the United States suffer from an autoimmune disease, and this number is increasing. Women are 75 percent more likely than men to have an autoimmune disease, especially in their childbearing years, and autoimmune diseases are one of the ten leading causes of death for women under the age of 65. If you have one autoimmune disease, you have a greater risk of developing another one, as well. There are more than 80 recognized autoimmune diseases and many more conditions and diseases that are suspected to be linked to an autoimmune response in the body. These diseases can affect almost every part of the body, and there is no cure.

The specific causes of autoimmune diseases are still largely a mystery, but we do know that genetics and environmental triggers play a role. Environmental factors could be anything that promotes inflammation, such as toxins, allergens, stress, and what we eat—the modern world is filled with potential triggers.

As little as 10 years ago, autoimmune diseases were not as prevalent. Researchers and medical professionals have not pinpointed the exact reason why there has been such a sharp increase in autoimmune diseases, but genetics cannot be the main trigger when these increases are so fast. This suggests that the environmental triggers present in everyday life, such as chemicals, pesticides, toxins, food additives, and heavy metals, play a role. If you add the chronic stress of modern life and other factors, such as hormones and genetic predisposition, you have a perfect storm in the immune system for the development of an autoimmune disease.

One avenue researchers have been studying is the link between autoimmune diseases and diet. The standard Western diet is full of chemicals, excess sugar, inflammatory foods, and trans fats. These eating habits set the stage for a condition called leaky gut, which is present in many who have an autoimmune disease. Dr. Alessio Fasano singles out intestinal permeability (leaky gut) as one of the three triggers that most likely causes autoimmune diseases.

Diets like the Autoimmune Paleo Diet are designed to heal leaky gut by eliminating foods that trigger an inflammatory response in the body. This Paleo-based elimination diet can reverse symptoms and, in some cases, put the disease in remission. A 2014 study published in the *Journal of Alternative and Complementary Medicine* looked at the effects of a modified Paleolithic diet and exercise routine on fatigue caused by multiple sclerosis and concluded that after one year there was a significant improvement of symptoms. This approach to treatment, addressing the cause rather than medicating the symptoms, is gaining popularity because it works at the root of the disease and it is in your control. Many people with an autoimmune disease feel their lives have spun out of control, so taking back control is critical to well-being.

The Autoimmune Paleo Diet can often help bring about a partial or significant remission of disease, which means your symptoms will be significantly reduced or temporarily healed. This temporary healing could last for years—and if you maintain a healing diet and watch other lifestyle triggers, remission could last the rest of your life. Remember that the gastrointestinal tract is not just where you digest food; it is the location of about 70 percent of your immune system, so it makes sense that diet is crucial to managing auto-immune diseases. Healing your gut will positively affect your whole body.

This book is structured to help you learn about autoimmune diseases and explore how diet and digestion affect the development and course of these diseases. We'll look at the possible effects of eliminating certain foods, the ingredients that will support your health, and lifestyle changes that should go hand in hand with the diet. This foundation will give you valuable knowledge about how your body works, so the diet itself will make perfect sense.

You'll also find detailed lists of foods to eliminate and why because it is easier to stop eating something when you understand the science behind the exclusion. There are lists of foods you can eat, too, as well as those that might be a gray area for you.

Part 2 outlines the action plan to heal your gut and ease your symptoms. A 30-day meal plan based on the more than 120 delectable recipes in part 3, along with easy-to-follow weekly shopping lists, take the guesswork out of the first month on the diet. You'll also learn how to reintroduce foods so you can successfully adjust your diet for the long haul.

Any elimination diet is challenging because you are removing familiar and loved foods from your meals, and this can be hard and downright scary.

The 30-day meal plan is designed to get you through the first month without having to think too much about what you need to cook or buy from the grocery store. The meal plans are flexible, and if you find a dish that you really like, feel free to repeat it whenever you want. The meal plan also introduces you to food seasoned with herbs and rich in flavor and texture, so you won't feel deprived. If you need to continue the elimination process for longer than 30 days, it will be easy for you to create your own meal plans or simply repeat the 30-day plan until you are symptom-free.

The Autoimmune Paleo Diet Cookbook gives you the tools to heal yourself through diet. You will learn:

- Why certain foods exacerbate intestinal permeability and increase the severity of your symptoms
- How to track your symptoms during both the elimination and reintroduction phases of the diet
- What to expect physically and emotionally when you start the diet
- Whether to take supplements and which ones
- Which lifestyle factors need to be managed so they don't negatively affect your disease
- How to cut the cost of your grocery bill and still enjoy delicious, nutritious meals
- How and when to reintroduce challenge foods safely
- How to troubleshoot your reactions to challenge foods
- More than 120 creative, nutritious recipes that will help you explore an eating plan that doesn't damage your body

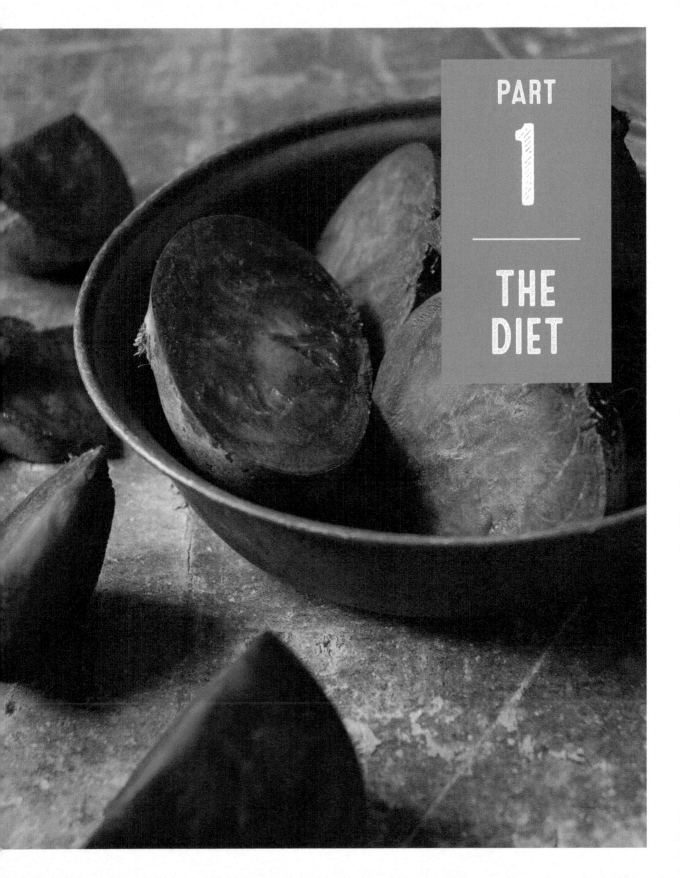

PART

1

THE
DIET

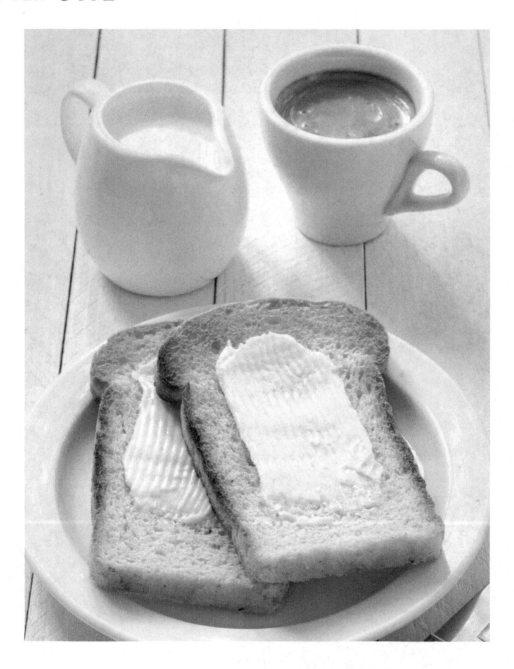

CHAPTER ONE

AUTOIMMUNE DISEASES AND YOUR DIET

According to estimates from the American Autoimmune Related Diseases Association (AARDA), autoimmune diseases are the number two cause of chronic illness in the United States, but less than 3 percent of the total budget for the National Institutes of Health (NIH) is dedicated to research into these diseases. This lack of knowledge about the causes, risk factors, and the best course of treatment raises questions for many people who live with autoimmune diseases every day.

One thing doctors and researchers do know is that inflammation plays a role in the development and severity of autoimmune diseases, so it makes sense to look at treatments that address inflammation. That's why many dieticians recommend an anti-inflammatory diet rich in nutrients. This approach reduces inflammation and corrects the vitamin deficiencies that are found in many autoimmune patients.

The question then is which diet to follow? The Autoimmune Paleo Diet meets all the parameters of an elimination diet designed to pinpoint trigger foods to help you manage and reduce the impact of an autoimmune disease on your life. The diet has been proven to work for many people, and studies of the links between diet and immunity seem to support it. Food does matter, and with your food choices, you have the ability to take control of your health and improve it.

An Autoimmune Disease Primer

Understanding autoimmune diseases and the factors that affect the severity of symptoms can be a positive first step to finding relief. Autoimmune diseases occur when the immune system, which is supposed to protect the body from bacteria, viruses, and other outside invaders, instead attacks the body. Which part is under attack will determine how the autoimmune disease manifests.

The immune system is composed of the tonsils, spleen, lymph nodes, bone marrow, and white blood cells, which work together to protect the body. When your immune system is healthy and functioning the way it is meant to, it can identify the cells that make you sick and target them for destruction. A healthy immune system does not mount an immune response against the cells of the body.

The white blood cells include monocytes and lymphocytes that can be further broken down into B cells, T cells, and natural killer cells. B cells produce antibodies (also known as immunoglobulins) to eliminate antigens, which are foreign bodies such as bacteria, cancer cells, viruses, and toxins. They do this by targeting particular proteins in the antigens. When the immune system identifies an antigen, specific antibodies released by the B cells bind to the invaders and signal the white blood cells to eliminate that antigen. If you come into contact with that antigen again, the immune system remembers it and the specific antibodies are produced to help destroy it. That's how immunizations work.

There are five types antibodies, and they work alone or in combination, depending on the threat to the body.

- **IgA:** These antibodies provide the ability to fight off antigens before they enter the bloodstream. They are found in the gut, respiratory system, breast milk, tears, and saliva.

- **IgD:** These antibodies act as antigen receptors and can activate other cells in the immune system. They are found on the cell membranes of B cells that have not been in contact with antigens.

- **IgE:** These antibodies cause the symptoms in an allergic response because they trigger a release of histamine when they bind with allergens.

- **IgG:** These antibodies provide a lifetime of protection against specific antigens and typically are the most numerous type of antibody, making up about 75 percent of our antibodies.

- **IgM:** These antibodies primarily protect the blood and are the first antibodies to appear, before adequate numbers of IgG are circulating to eliminate specific antigens.

When you're looking at autoimmune diseases, it's important to recognize the difference between autoimmunity and autoimmune disease. Autoimmunity is when the immune system mistakes the cells of the body for invaders and attacks them, and this occurs regularly. Sometimes the body makes autoantibodies, which mark the body's own proteins along with those of foreign invaders. This attack can occur anywhere in the body and affect many parts at once. It happens because some lymphocytes can react against the body, but this capability is usually suppressed. If the lymphocytes are not suppressed, an autoimmune response occurs. Low-level autoimmunity is normal and can actually be beneficial because it can prime the immune system to respond to a true threat, without causing damage to the body.

Having autoantibodies does not mean you will automatically develop an autoimmune disease, although it could be the first step. If the body fails to eliminate these autoantibodies and the cells producing them, the body will continue to attack itself because the immune system has been stimulated. As this process continues, the body will be damaged enough to show symptoms.

The area damaged and under attack determines the type of autoimmune disease. Autoimmune diseases can affect one area of tissue, specific organs, or the entire body. Because of this vast range of vulnerable areas, autoimmune diseases are often grouped by the body parts that are affected. The common groupings are:

Blood and blood vessels	Kidneys
Digestive tract	Lungs
Eyes and ears	Muscles
Glands	Nerves and brain
Heart	Skin
Joints	

The cause of autoimmune diseases is not completely understood by the medical community, but an interaction between genetics and environmental factors appears to play a role. Even if you have the genes that predispose you to autoimmune disease, you still might not develop it unless something in the environment triggers the autoimmune response in the body. Also, if autoimmune disease runs in your family, this does not mean you will get the same disease as your cousin or your parent.

The environmental factors related to autoimmune diseases account for more than half the risk factors. Known triggers include infections, drugs, hormones, viruses, bacteria, smoking, UV radiation, food, pollutants, and stress. Some of these factors cannot be controlled, but anything related to diet and lifestyle are within your power to influence positively.

The ten most common autoimmune diseases are:

1. Celiac disease (damages the lining of the small intestines)
2. Glomerulonephritis (attacks the small blood vessels in the kidneys that act as tiny filters)
3. Graves' disease (attacks the thyroid)
4. Hashimoto's thyroiditis (causes thyroid hormone deficiency)
5. Multiple sclerosis (attacks the protective coating around the nerves)
6. Pernicious anemia (the body fails to make enough healthy red blood cells)
7. Rheumatoid arthritis (attacks the lining of the joints throughout the body)
8. Systematic lupus erythematosus (damages the joints, skin, kidneys, heart, lungs, and other parts of the body)
9. Type 1 diabetes (attacks the cells that make insulin)
10. Vitiligo (destroys the cells that give the skin its color)

While these diseases can be diagnosed definitively, some kinds of autoimmune diseases are very difficult to diagnose because they present as an assortment of symptoms that often do not seem to be related to one another. These symptoms can be the signs of other physical concerns, as well, such as stress or lack of sleep. There is no definitive test for autoimmune diseases, so a diagnosis is often made using lab results such as blood tests and medical history to rule out other problems.

The challenge of getting a proper diagnosis is not the end of the obstacles, because there is no cure for autoimmune diseases. Standard medical treatment often involves replacing hormones or deficient vitamins, managing pain, and taking immunosuppressant drugs. Lifestyle and diet choices can also positively affect autoimmune diseases, which is why the Autoimmune Paleo Diet can help you take control of your health. Addressing diet issues while managing sleep, exercise, and stress can help your body heal and reduce the impact of an autoimmune disease on your life.

Have an Advocate for Support   Dealing with an assembly of doctors, nurses, specialists, and even pharmacists for your condition can be exhausting and stressful, and having a health advocate can help alleviate that stress. An advocate is someone who understands your needs and is knowledgeable about your condition and medical history. This person can take notes during appointments and make sure your treatment plan is respected. This type of support does not mean that you aren't in charge of your care, it means you have the added support of someone who understands your specific health goals.

Diet and Autoimmune Diseases

Diet is one of the environmental triggers associated with developing an autoimmune disease and the continued flare-up of symptoms that can occur. When you keep eating problem foods, they can irritate the lining of your gut, create inflammation, and feed the bacteria that naturally live in your body, causing overgrowth. Although diet is not the only cause of autoimmune diseases, it is one that is within your control, and you will see significant positive changes in your health when your diet is a solution, not a trigger.

Gluten

Although all the links between autoimmune diseases and diet are still unclear, it is understood that gluten plays a significant role. The reason is that gluten may be linked to a condition known as leaky gut, or intestinal permeability. The gut plays an important role in the immune system because it is one of the organs that is a boundary between the inside of the body and outside world. Intestinal permeability occurs when junctions in the gut that control what passes through the lining of the small intestine don't work properly. When that happens, substances can leak from the intestines into the bloodstream. This leakage can include pathogens, incomplete proteins, waste products, and even the friendly bacteria that is meant to stay in the gut.

For example, people with celiac disease and Crohn's disease (two autoimmune diseases of the gut) experience leaky gut. The body reacts to this influx of foreign material by creating an inflammatory response.

A leaky gut can develop over time and can be exacerbated by lifestyle factors such as medication, stress, and lack of sleep. Leaky gut is poorly understood, but some practitioners think it may have some connection to gluten, or more specifically a protein fraction of gluten called gliadin that in some people increases intestinal permeability. If so, eliminating grains and pseudograins (seeds and grasses that are commonly labeled as grains) can help heal the gut and even reverse a leaky gut over time.

Gut Microflora

We all have organisms living in our gut, much of which we need for a healthy life. There are approximately 100 trillion microorganisms living in the gut, made up of about 500 to 1,000 different species. Almost all are various species of bacteria. Different bacterial species prefer different microenvironments, so the ones in your colon might be different than the ones in the mucus lining of your small intestine. These microflora have a range of functions that are essential to ongoing good health, including breaking down nutrients, synthesizing vitamins, aiding in mineral absorption, and modulating the immune system by keeping some types of immune cells in check and stimulating others to produce antibodies.

This list of important functions means that a healthy, balanced microflora population is crucial to a healthy immune system. The composition of the microflora population is affected by your diet, because what you eat is also eaten by the microorganisms in the gut. For example, eating animals that have been treated with antibiotics can throw the microflora out of balance. Antibiotics do not only kill bad bacteria that can cause illness; these drugs also indiscriminately destroy good bacteria, including the microflora found in the gut, which can create an imbalance. In 2009 factory farms used over 29 million pounds of antibiotics, according to the Food and Drug Administration (FDA), and some of those antibiotics remained in the animal products we consumed. To avoid consuming antibiotics your body doesn't need, and to support healthy gut flora, choose organic meats untreated by antibiotics.

An abnormality in the gut's microflora is called gut dysbiosis. Gut dysbiosis accompanies many autoimmune diseases, in particular an overgrowth of yeast. Yeast feeds on refined carbohydrates, so a diet high in sugar and grain products can cause yeast to proliferate in the gut beyond normal levels.

Eliminating grains and some other hard-to-digest foods and eating organic meat can help restore the gut microflora to normal levels.

Hormones and Diet

Hormones can trigger an autoimmune disease, especially in women, which is why autoimmune diseases often manifest during puberty or pregnancy. Hormones are chemical messengers excreted into the blood, which carries them to organs and tissues. There, they regulate a wide variety of physical processes, including growth, metabolism, sexual function, and mood.

The sex hormones (estrogen, progesterone, and testosterone) can influence the immune system in many ways. Estrogen, in particular, can stimulate or suppress the immune system, while other hormones influence the effect of estrogen. This delicate system can easily be thrown out of balance. The influential role of estrogen on the immune system is still being studied, and its effects are not well understood. But researchers do know that symptoms of certain autoimmune diseases can increase in intensity or wane depending on what point a woman is at in her menstrual cycle.

It is important not to interfere with the body's delicate hormonal balance when promoting healing. This includes avoiding estrogen in the environment. Natural estrogens can be found in many foods, including flaxseed, corn, soy, nuts, seeds, legumes, and alfalfa as well as dairy or meat from animals that are treated with hormones. Limiting the exposure to estrogens in food can help heal the inflammation associated with autoimmune diseases.

Micronutrient Deficiencies

Vitamin and mineral deficiencies have conclusively been linked in a variety of studies to autoimmune diseases, as one such study on the impact of vitamin D deficiency on autoimmune rheumatic diseases proved in 2008 in *Arthritis Research and Therapy*. Micronutrient (nutrients we need in small amounts) deficiencies can be caused by absorption problems, where an impaired gut cannot absorb all the nutrients in what you eat. This may be the result of leaky gut or gut dysbiosis. Micronutrient deficiencies can also be caused by eating a nutrient-deficient diet.

Combining a diet high in refined carbohydrates and processed foods with a nutrient deficiency has a profound effect on the immune system. Processed foods are a perfect example of the type of product that feeds the body with calories but does not nourish it. Processing takes away many of the nutrients found in the original whole food and adds antinutrients—substances that impede the absorption of whatever nutrients are left.

Eating an abundance of grains, legumes, and dairy also creates a micro-nutrient deficiency, because these are not as nutrient dense as some other foods, such as dark leafy greens, grass-fed meat, and fish. You can eat only so much food per day, so it is important to maximize the amount of nutrients you consume. Replacing nutrient-dense foods such as vegetables, fruit, fish, seafood, and meat with these dietary lightweights deprives the body of essential vitamins, minerals, and phytonutrients (beneficial substances found only in plants).

Many people with autoimmune disease are deficient in micronutrients that help regulate the immune system. Some of the micronutrients that support healthy immunity are vitamins A, B_5, B_6, B_{12}, C, folic acid, E, and K as well as iron, zinc, copper, selenium, and manganese. A deficiency in these micro-nutrients can produce the following effects:

- Decreased blood lymphocyte counts
- Decreased production of antibodies from B cells
- Fewer antibodies circulating in the blood
- Impaired and suppressed T cell function
- Impaired normal antibody response
- More infections

Healing the body requires an abundance of micronutrients, so following a diet rich in nutrient-dense foods while eliminating foods that impede absorption or provide no nutritional value is vital in managing autoimmune diseases.

Other Dietary Factors

There are many other dietary factors that can positively or negatively affect autoimmune diseases. Since inflammation plays a key role in stimulating the immune response, eating a variety of foods containing inflammation-busting antioxidants, including vegetables and fruits, promotes healing. Eating quality saturated fat is also important because fat-soluble vitamins, such as vitamins A, D, E, and K, require fat to be absorbed and help regulate the immune system. Finding a diet that limits the exposure to foods that damage or disrupt the immune system and includes foods that support and heal the body is a sound strategy for managing and improving autoimmune diseases.

Why Paleo?

The basic Paleo diet provides a logical starting point for eliminating the foods that trigger a leaky gut. Grains, legumes, most dairy, processed vegetable oils, refined sugar, and processed foods are excluded from the diet. Instead, it focuses on meat, fish, seafood, poultry, eggs, vegetables, fruits, nuts, and seeds in their most natural, whole forms. Paleo is based on the diet of our ancestors before the advent of the agriculture, when people ate a diet that supported a healthy digestive system and did not cause harmful inflammation in the body.

The Paleo diet immediately addresses issues that are linked to a variety of food sensitivities, including wheat, gluten, and dairy, and can be a good place to start when you're considering a diet intervention for an autoimmune disease. It can be beneficial to try a strict Paleo diet first (before jumping into the Autoimmune Paleo Diet) to see if your symptoms and flare-ups subside, and then decide if you need further restrictions to find relief. This approach can ease you into the food choices, cooking requirements, and lifestyle changes that are required for a successful transition into a full Autoimmune Paleo Diet.

Food Sensitivity Testing   The Autoimmune Paleo diet can significantly improve the symptoms of your condition. However, if you are following the diet strictly, including the recommended reintroduction protocol, and your symptoms return or do not subside, then you might be sensitive to a food not included in the elimination list. If this is the case, food sensitivity testing could offer answers. ELISA testing is the most common test used to measure the level of immune reaction in the body to food proteins. Consult a qualified professional to determine which testing (IgE, IgG, or IgA) is right for you and be aware that these tests can sometimes offer false negatives or positives.

What Is the Autoimmune Paleo Diet?

The Autoimmune Paleo Diet is an elimination diet to help heal a leaky gut by pinpointing and avoiding foods that trigger symptoms of autoimmune diseases. In general, an elimination diet excludes all foods that might be potential triggers for an autoimmune response in the body. The Autoimmune Paleo Diet includes all the restrictions of the basic Paleo diet and also eliminates foods that have been linked to increased intestinal permeability or are common food intolerances for those with autoimmune diseases.

The Autoimmune Paleo Diet is meant to be followed until symptoms subside—typically for between 30 and 90 days, depending on the severity of your condition. Once you're feeling better, you reintroduce small amounts of some of the foods on the restricted list, one at a time, to gauge your body's reaction. Trying just one food at a time enables you to pinpoint exactly what your problem foods are. This reintroduction process can take time, but in the end you should have a clear understanding of which foods can safely be included in your regular diet again. There usually are some foods that never find their way back into the diet, and these include those that are also not allowed on the basic Paleo plan: grains, legumes, refined oils, refined sugar, and all processed foods.

FODMAPs (fermentable oligosaccharides, disaccharides, monosaccharides, and polyols) are a group of short-chain carbohydrates that some people cannot digest easily. Because they are hard to digest, the carbs are not absorbed completely in the small intestine. They then move through the digestive tract into the large intestine, where they ferment when digested by the gut's microflora. They also have an osmotic effect, which means they increase fluid movement into the large bowel. The combination of fermentation and osmosis causes bloating, gas, cramps, pain, diarrhea, and constipation for people who are sensitive to these foods. There are many common foods that are high in FODMAPs, including lactose from dairy products, fructose from certain fruit, coconut products, sweeteners, fructans from fibrous vegetables, and polyols from fruit and sugar alcohols.

You might have to adjust the Autoimmune Paleo Diet to reflect any additional food sensitivities or FODMAP issues you have. It is extremely important to listen to your body and tailor your diet to reflect your individual intolerances. If you know eggs are not a problem for you, eat them; if coconut milk causes you issues, substitute something else that does work for you.

Here are the basic Autoimmune Paleo Diet guidelines.

Permanently Eliminate

Emulsifiers and thickeners	Processed foods
Grains	Refined oils
Legumes	Refined sugar

Eliminate, Then Reintroduce (in Its Whole Form, if Possible)

Alcohol	Nuts, nut flours, nut oils, and nut butters
Cocoa	
Coffee	Seeds, seed flours, seed oils, and seed butters
Dairy	
Eggs	Spices derived from fruits
Nightshades	Spices derived from nightshades
Nonsteroidal anti-inflammatory drugs (NSAIDs)	Spices derived from seeds

Other Factors to Consider

- Choose grass-fed meat and organic products whenever possible
- Get a moderate amount of exercise daily
- Include probiotic and fermented foods, such as sauerkraut and kefir
- Include foods that are healing, such as bone broth, coconut oil, and organ meats
- Include nutritive sweeteners such as maple syrup and honey occasionally
- Limit fruit to two to five servings per day, and fructose (natural fruit sugar) to 20 grams per day
- Manage your stress
- Sleep at least eight to ten hours a day

What to Expect

Starting a diet that eliminates so many of the foods that make up a standard American diet can be daunting—both emotionally and physically. The most important aspect of the Autoimmune Paleo Diet is to start it and stick to it, so you can learn what strategies will enable you to heal yourself. If your current eating habits are drastically different from the Autoimmune Paleo Diet, though, your initial reaction to the diet might be negative rather than positive, and the severity and duration of your initial response to the diet will also vary. Know what to expect and stick it out. These reactions are all temporary—signs that your body is cleansing itself and starting to heal.

Some people dive right into the diet and follow it to the letter, while others transition slowly. No matter what your approach, you can expect to experience at least a few of the following side effects when you start. Treat them as signs that you are doing something right.

Cravings

Food cravings can be a serious issue for people switching to the Autoimmune Paleo Diet, for both physical and psychological reasons. Drinks like coffee are addictive due to the caffeine, so giving them up can create an intense reaction in the body. Also a large part of cravings is that many foods are a habit, like coffee while you read the morning paper, so changing routines can create a longing for the eliminated foods. Another aspect of food cravings is that many things, including food, seem more desirable when you can no longer have them. Eventually, you will create new habits, such as bone broth in the morning and a perfectly ripe piece of fruit for dessert instead of cake or cookies.

Detox Symptoms

If you transition from a Paleo diet (or another whole foods diet) to the Autoimmune Paleo Diet, you might not have any detox symptoms at all. However, if you eat a standard American diet filled with sugar, processed foods, and caffeine, you could experience headaches, fatigue, mood swings, and digestive problems. These symptoms happen when the toxins, preservatives, and other accumulated junk from a "regular" diet are flushed out. This detox reaction is a positive sign, because it means your body is cleaning out so it can start the healing process. Make sure you keep hydrated to help detoxification be quick and effective.

Digestive Problems

Digestion plays such a key role in the healing process for leaky gut that it makes sense you might have some digestive issues when starting the Auto-immune Paleo Diet. The digestive problems might include nausea, diarrhea, constipation, gas, bloating, and frequency of bowel movements. Some of these are symptoms you might have had before.

Many people have problems digesting fat, especially if they have had their gallbladder removed, but until they switch to a diet that is high in saturated fats perhaps the issue was not evident. Some of the digestion problems originate with the microflora present in the gut. When you change the foods you eat, you also alter the food source the microflora eats. This switch can drastically affect the population size, location, and diversity of the microflora, which in turn creates digestive upset as your body adjusts. Simply following the diet should clear up most of the digestive concerns, but if you are not seeing any improvement after a few weeks, consult your doctor.

Flu-Like Symptoms

This reaction to starting the Autoimmune Paleo Diet is sometimes known as the "low-carb flu." It is not a virus, though; it's just the symptoms of carb withdrawal. The headache, fatigue, weakness, mood swings, mental fog, and even joint or muscle pain can last for as long as a couple of weeks.

The severity of this reaction is linked to the amount of sugar and carbs you ordinarily eat. Most people who subsist on a carb-based diet have a metabolism fueled by sugar. Carbohydrates provide quick bursts of energy that cause sugar rushes and blood sugar crashes. When you cut out carbs and your body switches to a fat-burning metabolism, it takes time to get used to the change. This switch to a fat-burning metabolism provides a stable, slowing-burning source of energy that does not require you to eat constantly to avoid crashing. The low-carb flu will not last forever, so it is best just to ride it out and know that soon you will feel better.

The Jarisch-Herxheimer Reaction

As scary as it sounds, this is actually a very minor side effect in which your symptoms may appear to worsen for a day or two before they get better. The reaction is most often associated with antibiotic treatments but can also be connected to drastic changes in diet. When you change to a strict

Autoimmune Paleo Diet, it can cause the overgrowth of yeast in your gut to die off, releasing toxins as they do so, making you feel worse. Some of the symptoms of Jarisch-Herxheimer reaction are fever, nausea, headache, skin breakouts, chills, anxiety, muscle pain, and hyperventilation. If you don't have a yeast overgrowth, then you might not experience this reaction at all. If you do, the symptoms may last for only a few days at most, and it is just as likely that you won't experience any of these side effects at all.

Mental Fatigue

Information overload can be a genuine concern with the Autoimmune Paleo Diet. There is so much information on dietary and lifestyle recommendations that it can be difficult to commit to one course of action. One of the problems is that much of the available data seems to be contradictory, and there always seems to be a new study touting the benefits of a new superfood. Gathering the correct information about an autoimmune disease and applying it to your own health can be overwhelming.

It is important not to try everything all at once. Stressing over the "right" course of action is counterproductive. The Autoimmune Paleo Diet is a template for an eating plan that will work to heal your individual issues. It is not meant to be a one-size-fits-all solution, so tweak the food lists in any way that provides the greatest benefit to your body. The most important aspect of the plan is to follow your version consistently.

Weight Loss

Weight loss is often considered to be a positive response to a new diet, and it certainly might be if you need to lose some body fat. However, since many autoimmune diseases can cause weight loss due to digestive issues, you could have no weight to lose. One of the reasons you might experience weight loss is that many people do not replace the now forbidden carbohydrates with healthy fats, which creates a deficit in calories.

The main source of energy in the Autoimmune Paleo Diet comes from healthy fat, and it can be difficult for many people to overcome the diet prejudice concerning fat. For decades, saturated fats have been considered the pinnacle of dietary villains, so the initial weeks of the Autoimmune Paleo Diet might require an attitude switch. To combat unintentional weight loss, eat coconut oil, avocados, and leave the skin on your poultry.

Setbacks

There are very few people, if any, who can start an elimination diet and not have setbacks, both large and small. The Autoimmune Paleo Diet is not easy, even if you have been following a Paleo lifestyle for a while. One of the things to keep in mind, besides the goal of improving your health, is that this is not meant to be a permanent diet. Try to commit to the Autoimmune Paleo Diet for 30 days to track the changes in your body. If you do slip up and eat something that is not allowed, move on and try again. It would be beneficial also to take note of the circumstances and your emotional landscape surrounding the setback so that you can be aware of similar situations in the future.

Lack of Improvement

You should be prepared for the possibility that you might not see any improvement in the first few months of following the Autoimmune Paleo Diet. Your progress will depend on your inflammation level, the severity of your leaky gut, how much damage has already been done in your body, and even which cells are under attack. In some cases, the healing process can take years, although you should notice physical improvement along the way.

Do not give up if you do not experience a miracle cure from changing your diet. If you see no improvement at all after following the Autoimmune Paleo Diet strictly for three months, make sure that you are not sabotaging yourself with stress or lack of sleep. You can also discuss your progress with your doctor to see if you need to make further changes to deal with FODMAP considerations or add supplements to support the healing process.

Improvement in Symptoms and General Good Health

In as little as a couple of days to several weeks into the plan, you may well be feeling better and seeing tangible evidence that the elimination diet is working. Some people notice almost immediate improvement in their symptoms, depending on the severity of their condition when starting the Autoimmune Paleo Diet. You could enjoy deeper sleep, increased energy, and a reduction of migraines, mood swings, skin problems, joint pain, and breathing problems.

If you are feeling much better, it's still important to continue the elimination diet until all your symptoms subside completely, then follow the gradual reintroduction process. Pinpointing the foods that contribute to your autoimmune disease is crucial for your ongoing good health.

Lifestyle Overhaul Tips

- **Reduce stress.** Stress is a fact of daily life. Your body is designed to deal with acute bursts of stress to survive. If you had to run for your life, it is valuable to have an internal system in place to give you a little extra jump in your step. This is commonly called the fight-or-flight response, and cortisol and adrenaline work together to divert fuel to the brain and muscles from areas that are not crucial to immediate survival, such as digestion, reproduction, and the immune system.

   This response is perfect if the stressor is temporary, but low-grade chronic stress can create problems. Today, people are constantly under stress from work, traffic, home life, exercise, too much coffee, and too little sleep as well as bigger stressors such as the death of a loved one, divorce, and financial problems. With constant stress, the levels of cortisol in the body never have the opportunity to normalize, and this leads to chronic inflammation.

   The Autoimmune Paleo Diet will not be effective if you do not decrease the stress in your life. Ask for help at home with chores, learn to say no to too many commitments, spend some time outside, use your brain, and take a yoga or meditation class to learn how to quiet the endless monologue in your mind.

- **Get plenty of sleep.** Sleep is the key to healing yourself. Many important bodily functions occur when you sleep, including tissue repair. Sleep is crucial for regulating hormones, stimulating the immune system, and reducing inflammation in the body. A single missed night of sleep can raise the level of inflammation considerably. Chronic sleep deprivation, even losing one hour a night, can create real damage in the body and will even shorten your life.

   Unfortunately, the pain associated with some autoimmune diseases can disrupt sleep patterns. But as you move forward with a nutrient-packed diet, the symptoms of your autoimmune disease may subside enough to allow deep, healing sleep. Try to get at least eight to ten hours of sleep a night.

- **Safeguard your circadian rhythms.** Have you ever found yourself waking up at almost the same time every morning without an alarm clock? This is because you have an internal clock related to biological processes that occur roughly on a 24-hour schedule known as a circadian rhythm. This clock schedules body processes depending on what time of day it is, such as tissue repair at night and movement during the day. The time signals are passed through the body by increasing and decreasing the levels of certain hormones.

The immune system works on a circadian rhythm, as well, with the number of immune cells fluctuating depending on the time of day. Melatonin is one of the most important hormones that influence sleep, digestion, and the immune system. When your melatonin is thrown out of balance, you don't sleep as well, and abnormal levels of this hormone have been linked to flare-ups. Light and dark influence melatonin production, so make sure you get out in the sunshine during the day and use low-watt bulbs in your home at night.

- *Get moderate exercise.* Getting your body moving increases muscle mass, which boosts metabolism, reduces stress, promotes deep sleep, and improves bone density. Exercise also regulates hormones, including cortisol and melatonin, which positively affects the immune system.

  It is important to get the right kind of exercise when you are healing your body, because intense, long-duration cardio and high-impact training can stress the body and worsen the symptoms of most autoimmune diseases. Strenuous exercise can also cause leaky gut, because blood is diverted to the muscles and away from the gut. Moderate-intensity exercise is best for releasing a healthy level of cortisol and making sure your circadian rhythms aren't disrupted. Find something you enjoy, and get out and move your body.

  Take some vitamin D. Studies have shown that people with an autoimmune disease are more likely to be deficient in vitamin D, and several autoimmune diseases, such as multiple sclerosis, lupus, and type 1 diabetes, are more prevalent as you go farther from the equator. People closer to the equator are exposed to more sunshine in their daily lives, reducing the chance of vitamin D deficiency. According to a 2004 article published in the *American Journal of Clinical Nutrition*, a researcher found that if you have adequate levels of vitamin D in your body, your risk of developing an autoimmune disease seems to be less.

  The same researcher found that if you already have an autoimmune disease, taking vitamin D supplements or getting out in the sun (your body makes its own vitamin D when exposed to sunshine) can reduce the severity and duration of autoimmune flare-ups, particularly in patients with multiple sclerosis. This may be because vitamin D reduces the number of pro-inflammatory cytokines (proteins that serve as cell signalers), making it instrumental in the healthy functioning of the immune system. Along with safely basking in the sunshine, you can also eat foods rich in vitamin D, such as sardines and wild-caught salmon.

- *Gather support.* Having people who are there to encourage you and help along the journey to good health is invaluable. Sometimes even a hug from a loved one after a challenging day can be enough to reduce cortisol levels in the body and lower stress. Your family does not need to eat the Autoimmune Paleo Diet, although that would be convenient, but they can be supportive by not constantly tempting you with foods you can't eat. If your friends and family do not support what you are trying to achieve, then seek out like-minded communities either online or in your area. You can talk through the challenges and share your successes.

- *Consider your medications.* Going on the Autoimmune Paleo Diet does not mean you can stop taking your medications—although that might be an eventual goal, depending on your autoimmune disease, how long you've had the disease, and the damage done to your body. You should always discuss your medications with your doctor and decide together what an achievable goal is and whether your medications will impede healing. If you are going to change, taper off, or eliminate some medications altogether, it is important to do so under the supervision of a medical professional.

Autoimmune Disease FAQs

What kind of specialist treats people with autoimmune diseases?

Unlike other diseases that have specialists who concentrate on that particular ailment, such as a cardiologist treating heart disease, there are no autoimmune specialist doctors. The reason is that autoimmune diseases strike so many different parts of the body and present such a broad range of symptoms. If you have an autoimmune disease, you will be directed to a specialist who is an expert in the particular region of your body that is affected by the disease.

Some Medications That Can Interfere with Healing Your Gut

- Antibiotics used long term can kill off healthy microflora, which can create gut dysbiosis or overgrowth of harmful bacteria.

- Corticosteroids can relieve symptoms, but there are many side effects, such as sleep disruption, increased appetite, and fatigue.

- Disease-modifying antirheumatic drugs (DMARDs) are often used to treat auto-immune diseases, but they increase intestinal permeability; thus, paradoxically, a side effect of DMARDs is the risk of developing an autoimmune disease.

- Drugs that treat gastrointestinal problems (such as laxatives, antacids, and anti-diarrheal medications) can impede the absorption of nutrients and kill off healthy microflora in the gut.

- Hormone-based contraceptives influence the sex hormones, which can make managing autoimmune diseases difficult.

- NSAIDs can damage the gut barrier.

For example, if you have Graves' disease, you will see an endocrinologist, and if you have Celiac disease, you will be treated by a gastroenterologist.

Can you get only one autoimmune disease?

Unfortunately, if you have one autoimmune disease, you are at greater risk of developing another one. Having three or more autoimmune diseases is called multiple autoimmune syndrome. The reason could be genetic susceptibility or environmental factors, or both.

When you have more than one autoimmune disease, how do you know which symptoms are caused by which disease?

If you have two diseases that do not affect overlapping areas, this could be quite simple. If your autoimmune diseases cause similar symptoms, such as joint pain, or one or both of your autoimmune diseases are systemic in nature, then pinpointing the cause of a symptom could be quite difficult. Although it might seem important to know exactly which disease is flaring up, it is more valuable to find relief from the symptoms, and the treatment might be the same regardless.

Are autoimmune diseases contagious?

No. You can't catch an autoimmune disease, and it cannot be transferred to other people through blood or other fluids. The only time an autoimmune disease might be transferred from person to person is through pregnancy, and this is very rare. For example, a baby might be born with neonatal lupus if the mother has lupus.

What are flare-ups?

A flare-up is the serious sudden onset of your autoimmune disease symptoms. Autoimmune diseases fluctuate between flare-ups and periods of milder symptoms or remission. Flare-ups can be caused by many things, depending on your autoimmune disease. For example, cold weather can cause flare-ups if you have rheumatoid arthritis. It is important to pinpoint the reason for the flare-up so you can manage your disease and relieve the symptoms as quickly as possible. Some common reasons for flare-ups could be food, stress, or fatigue.

Are there holistic treatments that can help with autoimmune diseases?

The effectiveness of complementary and alternative medicine (also called holistic medicine) on autoimmune diseases is not a rich source of study. That makes it hard to determine if your particular autoimmune disease would be improved with holistic medicine such as herbal remedies, acupuncture, hypnosis, or massage. In any case, it is important to treat the underlying digestion problems rather than the symptoms of the autoimmune disease. Any holistic treatment should be discussed at length with your family health provider to ensure it does not interfere with any other therapies or medications.

Can an autoimmune disease affect fertility?

Women with autoimmune diseases can have difficulty getting pregnant, depending on their particular disease. The course of your pregnancy will be affected by the disease that you have, and symptoms could get better, stay the same, or worsen. Most women with autoimmune diseases can have babies safely, but there are risks linked to certain diseases. For example, women with myasthenia gravis can have trouble breathing while pregnant, and women with lupus have a higher risk of stillbirth. It is always advisable to discuss pregnancy plans with your family health professional before trying to get pregnant, learn about any risks associated with certain autoimmune diseases, and discuss any medication you might be taking to treat autoimmune diseases.

CHAPTER TWO

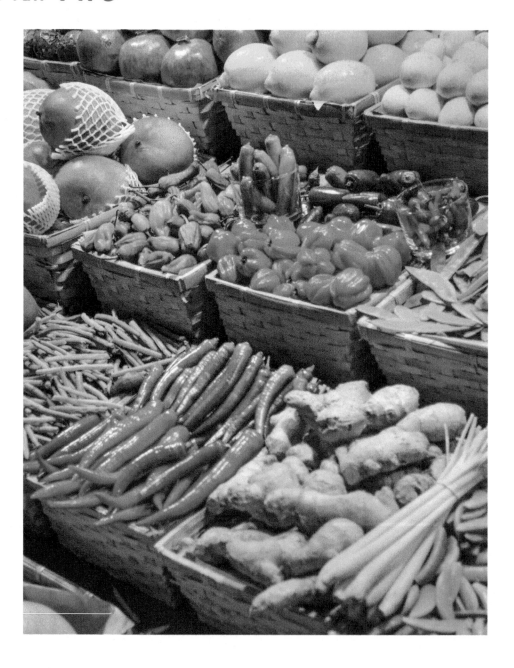

FOOD CHOICES

The guidelines of what foods should be eaten or avoided in this chapter are a framework for the basic Autoimmune Paleo Diet, but you can and absolutely should add those that don't affect you or subtract foods that do. Your Autoimmune Paleo Diet will be unique to you, so modify it as you see fit.

The list of approved foods is very diverse. Since these should always be whole foods with little or no processing, you can probably expect to spend more time and money on food while following the Autoimmune Paleo Diet. However, in the long run, the money you spend on quality ingredients to heal yourself may well be offset by savings in medical costs.

We cannot possibly list every food available, so pay attention to the families the foods fall under and add or avoid other foods in those families, as well. And remember that a general category like grain includes everything made from grain, such as bread, pasta, and cookies; soy includes soy sauce and tofu; and so on.

Foods, Drinks, and Medications to Avoid

Many diets have rules and do-not-eat lists that look very impressive, but sometimes it seems as if the science behind the recommendations is missing. Knowing why you are not supposed to eat something often makes it easier to resist the temptation. This information is particularly important when you are undertaking a plan designed to heal the body, like the Autoimmune Paleo Diet. The mechanics of what happens when you eat grains or have a glass of wine is crucial for understanding your own autoimmune disease and why you might experience flare-ups from egg yolks when someone else is not affected.

Alcohol

Alcohol can increase intestinal permeability in general and can increase the gut's permeability to toxins such as endotoxins and peptidoglycan, creating inflammation and an immune response. Drinking alcohol can also cause an overgrowth of pathogenic (gram-negative) bacteria because alcohol feeds this bacteria. Despite these issues, alcohol can sometimes be tolerated in limited amounts—about five ounces a week—as long as you stay away from grain-based alcohol and white wine, which can contain yeast that acts as a gluten cross-reactor.

Beans and Legumes

Beans and legumes are very similar to pseudograins in that they contain high levels of saponins and protease inhibitors. Saponins and protease inhibitors are linked to increased intestinal permeability. Legumes also contain lectins, which also can contribute to leaky gut.

There are many, many types of beans and legumes, including:

Adzuki bean	Fava bean	Navy bean
Alfalfa	Field pea	Peanut
Black bean	Great Northern bean	Pigeon pea
Black-eyed pea	Ground nut	Pinto bean
Butter bean	Kidney bean	Rooibos
Carob	Lentil	Runner bean
Chickpea	Lima bean	Soy
Clover	Mesquite	Split pea
Common bean	Mung bean	

Dairy Products

There are many reasons why dairy can affect anyone with an autoimmune disease and even people without any health problems. Milk contains lactose, a sugar that is not tolerated by about 25 percent of the population. Milk can alter the hormone levels in the body because it contains active bovine hormones. Hormone balance is crucial for an effective immune system. Dairy can contribute to leaky gut because it contains protease inhibitors and is pro-inflammatory. Eating dairy can increase mucus production, as well, creating issues with nutrient absorption in the gut.

Avoid anything with dairy in it (watch for milk in baked goods and other products not in the dairy family), including:

Butter	Frozen yogurt
Buttermilk	Ghee
Cheese	Ice cream
Cottage cheese	Milk kefir
Cream	Sour cream
Cream cheese	Whey
Curds	Whey isolate protein
Dairy protein isolates	Yogurt

Eggs

Although the entire egg is eliminated on the Autoimmune Paleo Diet, it is the egg white that typically causes the issue rather than the yolk. Some people with an autoimmune disease have no problems with the yolks. Egg whites are the defensive zone around the developing yolk. Egg whites contain proteins that are antimicrobial, and these proteins can create a negative reaction in people who have leaky gut. One of the proteins in egg whites can interfere with the absorption of biotin (a B vitamin), and another protein in the whites impedes the absorption of protein itself. A worse issue with egg whites is that some of the compounds present in them can move across the gut barrier and create further damage as well as an immune response.

Avoid all eggs and anything made with eggs, including baked goods.

Grains

Plants have natural defense systems that are designed to stop predators, such as people, from eating them. Part of this defense mechanism is a class of proteins called lectins. The structure of lectins cannot be broken down by the digestive enzymes found in humans, and since lectins contain protease inhibitors (enzymes that block the breakdown of protein), the digestive process is further obstructed. This lack of digestion means the lectins travel somewhat intact through the digestive system. Lectins then get passed through the enterocytes (intestinal absorptive cells) that line the gut by fooling the cells into thinking they are simple sugars. When the lectins pass out of the gut, they cause an inflammatory response, and this can damage or kill the enterocyte, inhibiting healthy digestion and creating a leaky gut.

All grains contain lectins, of which gluten is probably the best known. It can cause an incredible amount of damage in the body because its structure is very similar to other proteins in the body. This means that at least a few of the antibodies created to target gluten will also attack the normal cells of the body. These antibody attacks are part of the process that creates and increases the severity of an autoimmune disease.

Grains and grain products you are likely to come across include:

Barley	Rice
Bulgur (wheat groats)	Rye
Corn (maize)	Sorghum
Einkorn wheat	Spelt
Job's tears	Triticale
Kamut (Khorasan wheat)	Wheat
Millet	Wild rice
Oats	

Nightshades and Spices from Nightshades

All nightshade plants contain alkaloids, which protect them against insects by dissolving the insect's cell membranes and poisoning them. Alkaloids are toxic compounds and can affect humans, too. People with healthy immune and digestive systems can eat nightshades and have no reaction. People with autoimmune diseases are vulnerable to the effects of alkaloids; eating them can increase intestinal permeability and inflammation while overstimulating the immune system. Nightshades are also high in saponins, which are linked to increased gut permeability. The hotter, spicier nightshade peppers and spices contain gut-irritating capsicum, as well.

The foods in the nightshade family include:

Ashwagandha (Indian ginseng)	Chili pepper
Banana pepper	Chili pepper flakes
Bell pepper	Chili powder
Cayenne	Curry spice powder

Datil

Eggplant

Garam masala spice

Garden huckleberry

Goji berry (wolfberry)

Gooseberry (cape gooseberry, ground cherry)

Habanero

Jalapeño pepper

Jerusalem cherry

Naranjilla (lulo)

Paprika

Pepino

Pimento

Potato

Red pepper flakes

Tamarillo

Thai pepper

Tomatillo

Tomato

NSAIDs

NSAIDs can exacerbate leaky gut and be a gut irritator in general. Eliminating NSAIDs should be a personal decision, though, because many autoimmune diseases are characterized by excruciating pain that needs to be addressed. Pain is a stressful experience, and chronic pain can completely destroy healthy sleep patterns. Stress and lack of sleep can significantly worsen autoimmune diseases, so managing pain with NSAIDs might promote healing in the long run. If you need to manage pain associated with your autoimmune disease, discuss your options with your doctor to make the healthiest choice for you.

NSAIDs include:

Aspirin (Bayer, Excedrin)

Choline and magnesium salicylate (CMT, Tricosal)

Choline salicylate (Anthropan)

Celecoxib (Celebrex)

Diclofenac sodium (Voltaren, Voltaren XR)

Diflunisal (Dolobid)

Etodolac (Lodine, Lodine XL)

Fenoprofen (Nalfon, Nalfon 200)

Flurbiprofen (Ansaid)

Ibuprofen (Advil, Motrin, Motrin IB, Nuprin)

Ketoprofen (Actron, Orudis, Orudis KT, Oruvail)

Magnesium salicylate (Bayer Select, Mobidin)

Mefenamic acid (Ponstel)

Meloxicam (Mobic)

Nabumetone (Relafen)

Naproxen (Naprelan, Naprosyn)

Naproxen sodium (Aleve, Anaprox)

Oxaprozin (Daypro)

Rofecoxib (Vioxx)

Sodium salicylate (various generics)

Sulindac (Clinoril)

Tolmetin (Tolectin, Tolectin DS, Tolectin 600)

Valdecoxib (Bextra)

Nuts, Nut Oils, Nut Flours, and Nut Butters

Nuts and nut products have not been proven to cause increased intestinal permeability, but since this food group is the most common allergen after peanuts (a legume), it is advisable to remove all nuts during the elimination phase of the diet. People with autoimmune diseases are usually susceptible to allergies and sensitivities to foods such as nuts. Removing these foods can allow the gut to heal, and reintroducing nuts can pinpoint whether you have a problem. Similar to seeds, nuts are usually higher in omega-6 fatty acids rather than omega-3 fatty acids, and they also contain phytic acid and lectins.

Avoid nuts, oils made from nuts, and other nut products, including:

Acorn	Candlenut	Kola nut
Almond	Cashew	Macadamia
Beech	Chestnut	Pecan
Betel	Filbert	Pine nut
Black walnut	Ginkgo	Pistachio
Brazil nut	Hazelnut	Walnut
Butternut	Hickory	

Oils from Vegetables and Grains

These products are extracted using chemicals, which can leave behind a chemical residue. They are also very high in polyunsaturated fats and omega-6 fatty acids. Vegetable oils oxidize easily due to their polyunsaturated fat content, and this produces free radicals. Free radicals can increase inflammation in the body, and too much omega-6 fatty acid has also been shown to cause inflammation.

Oils you are likely to find include:

Canola oil	Grape seed oil	Shortening
Corn oil	Margarine	Soybean oil
Cottonseed oil	Palm kernel oil	Vegetable oil

Processed Foods

Processed foods are usually packed with ingredients that are not conducive to healing or recommended for good health in general. Processing strips food of nutrients and often adds ingredients that can impede the absorption of valuable vitamins and minerals. Preservatives, emulsifiers, thickeners, dyes, stabilizers, and antinutrients that are created during processing are harmful to the body. Antinutrients such as D-amino acids, lysinoalanine, oxidized sulfur amino acids, and additives such as guar gum, cellulose gum, xanthan gum, and lecithin impede the digestion of protein and minerals such as calcium, copper, and zinc. Guar gum and an additive called carrageenan have been linked to an increase in the severity of leaky gut in several studies, including one published in 1983 in the *Journal of Nutrition*.

Eliminate all processed foods, including emulsifiers, thickeners, and food additives.

Pseudograins

Pseudograins are the edible seeds of broadleaf plants; they resemble grains but are not in the same biological group. Pseudograins contain very high levels of compounds called saponins. Saponins are meant to prevent the plant from being eaten by insects and microbes. Saponins interact with cholesterol molecules that are found in cell membranes in the body, creating holes in the membranes. When these holes are created in the enterocytes that line the gut, the contents of the gut can leak through. These holes often kill the enterocyte cell and intestinal permeability increases along with inflammation in the body. Saponins also move through the holes created in the enterocytes and create problems in the bloodstream by destroying the membranes on red blood cells. This leakage creates further inflammation in the body.

Along with saponins, pseudograins also contain protease inhibitors. This is another plant defense that neutralizes the enzymes in the digestive tract so that they can't break down the protein in the plant into smaller amino acids. Consuming pseudograins prevents protein breakdown in the digestive tract, and this can cause the body to secrete more enzymes. This cycle can create an excess of some enzymes and a deficit of others. One enzyme that usually ends up in abundance is called trypsin, and this enzyme is particularly effective at breaking down connections between cells such as enterocytes. An excess of trypsin can contribute to leaky gut.

Pseudograins and products made from them that you are likely to come across include:

Amaranth	Chia	Quinoa
Buckwheat	Kañiwa	Teff

Seeds, Seed Oils, and Spices from Seeds

Seeds can increase inflammation in some people, but they are one of the foods that are removed from the Autoimmune Paleo Diet because they might cause problems, not because they definitely cause problems. Seeds are a source of lectins and phytic acid, both of which can increase intestinal permeability and interfere with the absorption of minerals. Seeds are also high omega-6 fatty acids, which can throw off the desirable ratio of omega-3 fatty acids to omega-6 fatty acids. Omega-6 fatty acids are pro-inflammatory, which means they increase inflammation, and omega-3 fatty acids are anti-inflammatory. A desirable ratio of these fatty acids means eating more omega-3 fatty acids than omega-6s, so that the net result does not produce inflammation.

Avoid seeds, oils made from seeds, and spices that are actually seeds, including:

Anise	Black mustard	Chia
Annatto	Caraway	Cocoa
Black caraway	Celery seed	Coffee

Coriander	Hemp	Rapeseed
Cumin	India mustard	Safflower
Dill	Mustard	Sesame
Fennel seed	Nutmeg	Sunflower
Fenugreek	Poppy	
Flax	Pumpkin	

Spices Made from Fruit

The spices that are derived from fruits are often mostly the seeds, which create issues associated with seed consumption. These spices are more on a "proceed with caution" list than a full exclusion list, but it is a good strategy to eliminate them at least for the first 30 days of the Autoimmune Paleo Diet.

Spices that are actually the fruit of the plant include:

Allspice	Green peppercorn	Star anise
Black peppercorn	Juniper	Vanilla bean
Cardamom	Pink peppercorn	White pepper

Sweeteners, Sugar Alcohols, and Sugars

Sugar can cause several different issues when you have an autoimmune disease, and refined sweeteners are particularly damaging. Sugar, sweeteners, and sugar alcohol can all irritate the gut and cause stress in the body. That's because these refined sugar products are completely depleted of minerals and vitamins. The body has to leech these nutrients from its own cells and tissues to metabolize the sugar. This drain on the body is damaging. Bacteria and yeast love to eat sugar, too, so including sweeteners in your diet can cause an overgrowth that contributes to gut dysbiosis.

Avoid both natural and artificial sweeteners, including:

Acesulfame potassium	Brown rice syrup
Agave	Brown sugar
Agave nectar	Cane (crystals, sugar, and juice)
Aspartame	Caramel
Barley malt and syrup	Coconut sugar
Beet sugar	Corn syrup

Date sugar

Demerara sugar

Dextrin

Dextrose

Erythritol

Fructose

Galactose

Glucose

Golden syrup

High-fructose corn syrup

Invert sugar

Lactose

Maltodextrin

Maltose

Malt syrup

Mannitol

Muscovado sugar

Neotame

Palm sugar

Raw sugar

Refined sugar

Rice bran syrup

Saccharin

Saccharose

Sorbitol

Sorghum syrup

Stevia

Sucanat

Sucralose

Sucrose

Sugar

Syrup

Treacle

Turbinado sugar

Xylitol

What About Supplements?

Supplements can be tricky when you are following the Autoimmune Paleo Diet. Vitamin or mineral supplements can be harmful if your diet is not in balance. For example, too much calcium can interfere with the absorption of iron, magnesium, and amino acids. Nutrients are also meant to work together in the body, along with fat, fiber, and protein. Eating a wide variety of nutrient-dense foods creates the correct combination and balance of nutrients required to heal autoimmune diseases.

Considering that digestive issues play such a huge role in autoimmune diseases, it is unlikely that supplements would be digested and absorbed in the gut any better than actual food. A whole foods diet is the best way to get all the nutrients your body needs, so your focus should be on food first, before you think about supplements.

That being said, there are many supplements that are advertised to support gut health or particular organs, treat specific aspects of your autoimmune disease, or address chronic infections, parasites, and overgrowth of bacteria or yeast. L-glutamine and deglycyrrhizinated licorice (DGL) can improve gut barrier function, magnesium and vitamin C are good for stress management, and fish oil can help the body absorb fat-soluble vitamins and vitamin D.

When using supplements, keep in mind these basic guidelines.

- Consult a health care professional before including any supplements in your diet.

- Read the labels on your supplements, because common fillers can contain gluten, dairy, or soy.

- Listen to your body and understand that your supplement needs will change as your gut heals and symptoms subside.

- Make sure the vitamins and minerals you take are in a form that is available to the body. This type of information should be available online or with a call to the manufacturer.

- Research the source of the supplement to ensure that organic ingredients that are not genetically modified (non-GMO) are used to make the finished product.

- Try one supplement at a time to gauge its effectiveness. Overwhelming a healing body with an assortment of supplements can be counterproductive.

- Be aware that your supplement and healing needs will be completely individual, so following a plan that is successful for someone else might not work for you.

All Things in Moderation

These gray-area foods should be fine either in moderation, which means don't eat them every day, or occasionally, which means don't eat them every week. The foods that can be eaten in moderation or occasionally depend on your individual reaction. For example, some of these foods contain caffeine, which can be an issue for some people, while others might not be able to tolerate nutritive sweeteners like maple syrup or honey. If you do add a sweetener, it is important to read labels to make sure it does not contain fillers, such as high-fructose corn syrup.

In Moderation

Apple cider vinegar

Black tea

Carob

Coconut products (coconut butter, creamed coconut, coconut flakes, fresh coconut)

Coconut water

Gluten-free balsamic vinegar

Green tea

Pomegranate molasses

Rooibos tea

Vanilla extract (cooked)

Wine vinegar

Occasionally

Date

Date sugar

Dried fruit

Honey

Maple sugar

Maple syrup

Molasses

Unrefined cane sugar

Check Your Reaction and Adjust Your Diet Accordingly

Egg yolk

Gluten-free alcohol

Grass-fed ghee

Macadamia nut oil

Peas with edible pods, eaten raw (green bean, snap pea, snow pea)

Walnut oil

Foods and Drinks to Include

You might be wondering what you will be eating now that you have seen the list of eliminated foods. You will be filling your plate with a colorful array of vegetables and fruits, organic meats and poultry, fresh fish and seafood, healthy fats, fragrant herbs, and fermented foods. There are so many tempting and delicious ingredients available to you that you will probably never get bored trying all of them.

Beverages

Carbonated water

Coconut milk

Coconut milk kefir

Coconut water

Herbal tea (with Autoimmune Paleo Diet–approved herbs)

Kombucha

Juices (fresh, made with Autoimmune Paleo Diet fruits and vegetables)

Lemon juice

Lime juice

Vegetable kvasses

Water

Water kefir

Fish

Anchovy	Gar	Monkfish	Salmon
Bass	Grouper	Orange roughy	Sardine
Bonito	Haddock		Snapper
Carp	Halibut	Perch	Sole
Catfish	Herring	Pickerel	Tilapia
Char	John Dory	Pike	Trout
Cod	Ling	Pollack	Tuna
Conger	Mackerel	Red snapper	Turbot
Eel	Mahi mahi	Rockfish	

Fruits

Cacti and other succulents
Cereus peruvianus
Dragon fruit
Citrus fruits
Blood orange
Citron
Clementine
Grapefruit
Kaffir lime
Key lime
Kumquat
Lemon
Limetta
Mandarin
Meyer lemon
Naartjie
Orange
Orangelo
Persian lime
Pomelo
Prickly pear
Rangpur
Saguaro
Sweet lemon
Tangelo
Tangerine
Ugli
Yuzu

Melons

Bitter melon
Canary melon
Cantaloupe
Casaba
Galia
Honeydew
Horned melon
Melon pear
Muskmelon
Persian melon
Watermelon
Winter melon

Temperate Fruits and Berries

Apple
Apricot
Bearberry
Bilberry
Blackberry
Black cherry
Black mulberry
Blueberry
Boysenberry
Chokeberry
Chokecherry
Cloudberry
Cornelian cherry
Crab apple
Cranberry
Crowberry
Currant
Dewberry
Elderberry
Falberry
Grape
Greengage plum
Hackberry
Hawthorn
Honeysuckle
Huckleberry
Jujube
Lingonberry
Loganberry
Loquat
Mayapple
Medlar
Mulberry
Nannyberry
Nectarine
Oregon grape
Papaw
Peach
Pear

Plum

Plumcot

Pomegranate

Quince

Raspberry

Rose hip

Rowan

Salmonberry

Sea-buckthorn

Serviceberry

Shipova

Sour cherry

Sweet cherry

Sycamore fig

Tayberry

Thimbleberry

Wineberry

Wolfberry

Tropical Fruits

Abiu

Acai

Acerola

Ackee

African cherry
  orange

African Moringa

Agave

Ambarella

American
  persimmon

Avocado

Babaco

Banana

Barbados cherry

Biriba

Black mulberry

Bolivian coconut

Burmese grape

Camucamu

Canistel

Carob

Cattley guava

Chayote

Cherimoya

Chilean guava

Chinese olive

Coco plum

Coconut

Costa Rican guava

Custard apple

Damson plum

Date

Date plum

Dragon fruit

Durian

Fig

Gambooge

Guanabana

Guava

Guavaberry

Indian fig

Indian jujube

Jackfruit

Jambool

Kiwifruit

Limeberry

Limequat

Longan

Lychee

Malabar plum

Malay apple

Mango

Mangosteen

Manila tamarind

Maypop

Meiwa kumquat

Melon pear

Miracle fruit

Nagami kumquat

Nance

Neem

Oriental persimmon

Papaya

Passion fruit

Persimmon

Pineapple

Pineapple guava

Plantain

Pomegranate

Pomelo

Pond apple

Purple guava
Rambutan
Riberry
Rose apple
Safou

Salak
Santol
Spanish lime
Star apple
Star fruit

Strawberry guava
Strawberry pear
Sugar apple
Tahitian apple
Tamarind

Herbs and Spices

Basil
Bay leaf
Chamomile
Chervil
Chives
Cilantro
Cinnamon
Clove
Garlic
Ginger
Horseradish

Lavender
Lemon balm
Lemongrass
Lime leaves
Mace
Marjoram
Onion (plus powder
   or flakes)
Oregano
Parsley
Peppermint

Rosemary
Saffron
Sage
Salt
Savory
Spearmint
Tarragon
Thyme
Turmeric
Wasabi

Meat

Bear
Beaver
Beef
Bison
Boar
Camel
Caribou

Deer
Elk
Goat
Kangaroo
Lamb
Moose
Mutton

Pork
Rabbit
Reindeer
Sheep
Turkey
Veal
Wild Boar

Offal and Body Parts

Blood

Bone

Brain

Chitterlings

Fat

Feet

Gelatin

Gizzard

Head meat

Heart

Kidney

Lips

Liver

Rinds

Sweetbreads

Tail

Testicle

Tongue

Tripe

Oils and Fats

Avocado oil

Bacon fat

Chicken fat

Coconut oil

Duck fat

Goose fat

Lard

Olive oil

Palm oil (but not palm kernel oil)

Tallow

Pantry Items

Agar

Arrowroot powder

Baking soda

Capers

Carob powder

Coconut aminos

Cream of tartar

Fish sauce (check ingredients)

Gelatin

Kudzu starch

Plantain flour

Tapioca starch

Truffle oil

Poultry

Chicken

Cornish hen

Dove

Duck

Emu

Goose

Grouse

Guinea hen

Ostrich

Partridge

Pheasant

Pigeon

Ptarmigan

Quail

Turkey

Nutrient Density

The Autoimmune Paleo Diet is focused on eliminating foods that damage the gut and understanding how those trigger foods affect the body. The second, equally important aspect of the Autoimmune Paleo Diet concerns the foods that you will be enjoying on the plan. You need to replace inflammatory foods with the most nutrient-dense foods possible to provide the variety and nutrition required by your body to heal.

Nutrient-dense foods are not necessarily the most expensive foods, but rather the highest quality you can afford in every category of food, from grass-fed, pasture-raised animals to organic produce. You need nutrient-dense foods to fix the micronutrient deficiencies that most people suffer from when eating the standard American diet and to provide the flood of nutrients you need to heal your gut and clear up inflammation.

Nutrient-dense foods pack the most vitamins, minerals, phytochemicals, and antioxidants into the fewest number of calories. There is a limit to the amount of food you can or should eat in one day, so it's important to maximize the benefit you receive from your choices.

Grass-fed, pasture-raised meat: These animals are raised eating grass their entire lives and, in an ideal situation, walking around in pastures. These animals are also not given antibiotics or hormones. Don't confuse organic meat with grass-fed, pasture-raised meat because they are not the same. Grass-fed animals can certainly be organic, but some organically raised animals are not grass-fed, so it is important to research the source of your meat. Chickens, pigs, and turkeys sometimes have their diet supplemented because they are not strict herbivores. Whenever possible, ask about what extra food is given to the animals so you can make an informed choice.

Grass-fed, pasture-raised animals provide a more nutrient-dense meat than those conventionally raised, although the actual difference will vary from species to species and farm to farm. In most cases grass-fed, pasture-raised meat is higher in minerals, vitamins, and antioxidants and has a healthier omega-6 fatty acid to omega-3 fatty acid ratio. Since the animals spend a great deal of time walking around in the sunshine, their fat is often a better source of vitamin D. The meat is usually leaner, has less water content, and tastes better.

Wild-caught fish and seafood: The nutritional difference between wild-caught and farm-raised fish is not as big a gap as with beef, chickens, and pigs. Regardless of where the fish is raised, it is still a fabulous source of omega-3 fatty acids, except for a few cases—farm-raised tilapia and catfish as well as freshwater bass are high in omega-6 fatty acids, too. Choose wild-caught salmon when you can because it is higher in nutrients and has a healthier omega-6 to omega-3 ratio than farm-raised salmon.

Offal: Eating the entire cow or pig with very little waste is ecologically sound and provides a great deal of nutrition. The organs of the animal are the most nutrient-dense part and are a valuable source of amino acids, collagen, and elastin. For example, the liver is an incredible source of vitamins A and D, iron, and copper. It might take you some time to get used to eating all the edible byproducts in your daily meals, but in the interest of healing, try to include offal in your diet two to four times a week.

Organic fruits and vegetables: On the Autoimmune Paleo Diet, you can eat unlimited amounts of vegetables and two to five portions of fruit per day (less than 20 grams of fructose), so it is crucial to find the best-quality produce you can afford. Produce is a rich source of vitamins, minerals, antioxidants, and phytonutrients, and if you eat a broad range of colorful choices, you will ensure all your nutrient bases are covered.

Buying organic produce is certainly a better choice, because you avoid all the toxins in pesticides that can be sprayed on produce. But if it is not possible, then at least go organic for the most contaminated produce, as outlined by the Dirty Dozen list (see the Appendix, page 276), to cut your risk of pesticide exposure. Organic produce is also, on average, more nutrient-dense than conventionally farmed products because industrial farming strips nutrients out of the soil, so food grown in the depleted soil does not absorb as many nutrients.

If you have diabetes or metabolic disease or are insulin-resistant, make sure you stick to low-glycemic fruits (fruits that do not rapidly raise your blood sugar, such as plums, cherries, apples, and kiwis) so your blood sugar is not thrown out of balance. Most fruit has a low-glycemic load, so if you stay within the portion recommendations, you should be fine.

Probiotic and Fermented Foods

Coconut kefir	Kombucha (without additives or extra sugar or thickeners)	Water kefir
Coconut kefir yogurt		
Fermented kimchi		
Fermented sauerkraut	Kvasses	

Reptiles and Amphibians

Alligator	Frog	Turtle
Crocodile	Snake	

Shellfish

Abalone	Lobster	Scallop
Clam	Mussel	Shrimp
Cockle	Octopus	Snail
Crab	Oyster	Squid
Crawfish	Periwinkle	
Cuttlefish	Prawns	

Vegetables

Alliums

Garlic	Shallot	Welsh onion
Leek	Spring onion (scallion)	Wild garlic
Onion		

Flowers, Stems, and Flower Buds

Artichoke	Caper	Rhubarb
Asparagus	Cauliflower	Squash blossom
Broccoli	Celery	Zucchini flower
Broccolini flower	Florence fennel	

Leafy Green Vegetables

Amaranthus	Broccoli rabe	Celery
Arugula (rocket)	Brussels sprout	Chickweed
Borage greens	Cabbage (all types)	Chicory
Broccoli	Cauliflower	Chinese cabbage

Collard greens

Cress

Dandelion

Endive

Fiddlehead

Grape leaves

Kale

Komatsuna

Lamb's lettuce

Land cress

Lettuce

Mizuna greens

Mustards, oriental

Napa cabbage

Nori

Radicchio

Sea lettuce

Seaweed

Sorrel

Spinach

Squash blossom

Swiss chard

Tatsoi

Turnip greens

Wakame

Watercress

FODMAP Foods

Foods high in FODMAPs may cause problems for some people on the Autoimmune Paleo Diet. FODMAPs are fructose, lactose, fructans, galactans, and polyols. So in addition to following the food lists for the Autoimmune Paleo Diet, if you are sensitive to FODMAPs, you might have to adjust your diet to reduce or eliminate the following.

Eliminate

Apple	Cherry	Leeks	Pears
Apricot	Chicory	Lychee	Persimmon
Artichoke	Dried fruit	Mango	Plum
Asparagus	Fennel	Mushroom	Shallot
Beet	Fruit juice	Nectarine	Snow pea
Blackberry	Garlic	Okra	Sugar snap pea
Cabbage	Jerusalem	Onion	Radicchio
Cauliflower	artichoke	Peach	Watermelon

Reduce Until You Know Your Reaction

Avocado	Butternut squash	Grape	Pumpkin
Beet	Cauliflower	Longan	Rambutan
Broccoli	Celery	Lychee	Sauerkraut
Brussels sprout	Fennel bulb	Mushroom	Sweet potato

Root Vegetables

Arrowroot	Daikon	Radish
Bamboo shoot	Ginger	Rutabaga
Beet	Horseradish	Salsify
Burdock	Jerusalem artichoke	Sweet potato
Carrots	Jicama	Taro
Cassava (yucca)	Kohlrabi	Turnip
Celeriac	Lotus root	Yam
Chinese artichoke	Parsnip	

Vegetables That Are Really Fruits

Avocado	Ivy gourd	Squash
Bitter melon (bitter gourd)	Luffa	Tinda
	Olives	West Indian gherkin
Chayote	Plantain	Winter melon
Cucumber	Pumpkin	Zucchini (courgette)

Trying Offal in Your Meals   Eating a nutrient-dense diet is the foundation of the Autoimmune Paleo plan, so including organ meats (offal) in your meals is a good idea. Most people shy away from consuming these unfamiliar cuts, but considering the relatively inexpensive cost and nutrition density of liver, heart, kidney, and other organ meats, you might want to try them. Keep in mind that organ meats from different animals taste different, so if you hate beef liver that does not mean chicken liver is also not palatable. Organ meats are similar to any other unfamiliar ingredient, experimentation with cooking techniques and accompanying flavors can create new favorites.

Produce for All Seasons

It is a good strategy to buy foods that are in season and grown locally when possible. First of all, they are usually cheaper than fruits and vegetables that have been shipped across continents. More importantly, most seasonal produce tastes better and is more nutritious because it is picked when it's almost ripe or ripe, rather than ripened chemically en route or in a storage facility. Furthermore, local produce usually is not treated with preservatives such as wax. In most places, you can find an incredible variety of seasonal produce to choose from. Obviously, the list of what is seasonal will change depending on where you live. This is not a comprehensive list for North America, but it is a good place to start.

Spring

Apricot	Chives	Lime	Spinach
Artichoke	Collard greens	Mango	Strawberry
Arugula	Fennel	Oranges	Vidalia onion
Asparagus	Fiddlehead	Pineapple	Watercress
Belgium endive	Grapefruit	Radicchio	
Broccoli	Honeydew	Red leaf lettuce	
Cauliflower	Jicama	Rhubarb	

Summer

Apricot	Cantaloupe	Loganberry	Red leaf lettuce
Arugula	Cherry	Nectarine	Strawberry
Asian pear	Cucumber	Okra	Summer squash
Beet	Elderberry	Passion fruit	Swiss chard
Blackberry	Endive	Peach	Zucchini
Black currant	Fig	Pineapple	Watermelon
Blueberry	Grape	Plum	▶
Boysenberry	Honeydew	Radish	
Broccoli	Limes	Raspberry	

Produce for All Seasons *continued*

Fall

Acorn squash	Butter lettuce	Kale	Quince
Apple	Butternut squash	Kohlrabi	Radicchio
Arugula	Cauliflower	Kumquat	Radish
Asian pear	Cranberry	Passion fruit	Sweet potato
Belgium endive	Endive	Pear	Swiss chard
Broccoli	Grape	Pomegranate	Winter squash
Brussels sprout	Jicama	Pumpkin	

Winter

Acorn squash	Clementine	Kale	Pineapple
Belgium endive	Collard greens	Kiwi	Pomegranate
Brussels sprout	Date	Orange	Sweet potato
Butternut squash	Grapefruit	Passion fruit	Tangerine
Cauliflower	Jicama	Pear	Winter squash

Year-Round

Avocado	Cabbage	Lemon	Parsnip
Banana	Carrot	Lettuce	Shallot
Beet greens	Celery	Mushroom	Turnip
Bok choy	Celeriac	Onion	
Broccolini	Leek	Papaya	

Food FAQs

Can you jump into the Autoimmune Paleo Diet?

The best way to start this diet is to make a plan and be aware of exactly what you need to do with your food and other lifestyle changes. Part 2 of this book will guide you through that process. Do as much homework as possible before embarking on this diet, and have a clear goal in mind. You will be on the diet for at least 30 days and possibly longer depending on the severity of your condition, so try to start during a relatively calm period of your life. Huge social events, stressful life changes such as moving, and projects at work can all draw your energies away from the diet. Obviously, life does have a way of being busy, so don't wait forever to start the Autoimmune Paleo Diet, especially if your symptoms are aggressive.

Can you cheat on the Autoimmune Paleo Diet?

If you mean eating a stack of buttermilk pancakes slathered in butter, whipped cream, and syrup, then no. If you want to try eating an egg yolk after following the diet for a few weeks, it might be fine. In the best-case scenario, you will follow a strict Autoimmune Paleo Diet until your symptoms subside, excluding the foods that are recommended and eating the gray-area foods only in moderation or as a snack. This plan is not meant to be followed for the rest of your life, but cheating with trigger foods while you are trying to heal will only set your health back. That plate of pancakes might not seem as appetizing when you consider that it might take months to calm your physical reaction. Keep in mind that if you follow the diet and reintroduction phase as they are outlined in part 2, you might find that butter, eggs, chocolate, and some types of nuts have no effect on you, and you can enjoy these foods as part of your regular diet.

Do you have to start on day one again if you cheat?

Yes. The way the Autoimmune Paleo Diet works is based on avoiding the foods on the elimination list for a minimum of 30 consecutive days, so that your body can heal and so you can track any responses to foods you add after that point. If you do fall off the Autoimmune Paleo Diet wagon, just start again. You will eventually reach the point where you can try foods again.

Why does the body react so strongly to foods after being on the Autoimmune Paleo Diet?

Before following the Autoimmune Paleo Diet you were probably eating many foods to which you were intolerant, so your body was constantly suffering from inflammation. Eating a bit more of the food wouldn't cause a strong reaction because your symptoms were already present. When you follow the Autoimmune Paleo Diet until your body is healed and your symptoms subside, your body is free of the chronic inflammation that comes from eating foods that trigger an immune response. This means you will have an acute response if you eat a food that is a trigger. It obviously will feel awful, but this type of strong reaction is positive because it means the elimination diet is doing exactly what it is meant to do and you know to avoid that food in the future.

Isn't it easier just to get tests to pinpoint food sensitivities?

There are tests that are designed to tell you if certain foods are a problem for you. This can be useful information to have even if you are planning to follow the Autoimmune Paleo Diet, because some allowed foods could cause reactions in certain individuals. Allergy testing does not cover every food, though, so an elimination diet could be more beneficial to pinpoint triggers. Test results are not the whole story for many people, either, because ingredients that can affect the body negatively might not be a full-blown allergy.

Can you use fresh juices as meal replacements on the Autoimmune Paleo Diet?

No, juicing should not be used as full meal replacements because juices lack vital protein and fat. But fresh juices can be a supplemental part of the Autoimmune Paleo Diet. For example, have a glass of vegetable juice with a chicken patty or a homemade sausage for breakfast. Make sure you use Autoimmune Paleo Diet–approved fruits and vegetables and do not overload on high-fructose ingredients.

Does the Autoimmune Paleo Diet cause weight loss?

Whether you lose weight, maintain your current weight, or even gain weight will depend entirely on your physical condition before starting the diet. If you have not been paying close attention to your diet and eating a lot of processed foods, breads, and dairy, you might find yourself losing weight when these calorie-dense, low-nutrition foods are removed from your diet. Some autoimmune diseases cause weight loss due to digestion issues, so it is important for those who are underweight to not lose too much weight when starting the Autoimmune Paleo Diet. If you are underweight, include coconut, avocado, and other fat-rich foods to your diet daily. As your gut heals, you might find that your weight-loss problem goes away, and then you can scale back your fat consumption to maintain a healthy weight.

Are small, frequent meals the best strategy when following the Autoimmune Paleo Diet?

You should try to eat three satisfying meals a day and a snack rather than grazing. Each meal should include protein, healthy fat, and carbohydrates to maintain a balanced flow of nutrients throughout the day. If you cannot handle digesting large quantities of food all at once due to a damaged gut, break your meals up a little more to avoid any discomfort. Try not to eat within two hours of bedtime, though, because a full stomach can disrupt sleep.

Can a vegan follow the Autoimmune Paleo Diet?

It is not possible to get all the nutrients and micronutrients required to successfully heal a leaky gut and combat an autoimmune disease solely from plant-based foods. If you are mostly a vegetarian who still consumes fish and seafood, the diet could be successful, if you follow a very well-thought-out meal plan.

Do you have to eat a great deal of meat on the Autoimmune Paleo Diet?

Healthy meats, poultry, fish, and seafood are the foundation of the Paleo diet and also play an important role in the Autoimmune Paleo Diet. Lean meats are a rich source of protein, B vitamins, magnesium, zinc, and iron. Adults usually require at least 60 to 80 grams of protein a day, which is about three servings or 10 ounces. Getting adequate protein can boost the immune system and help the body fight off infection and disease while promoting a healthy cardiovascular system and nervous system.

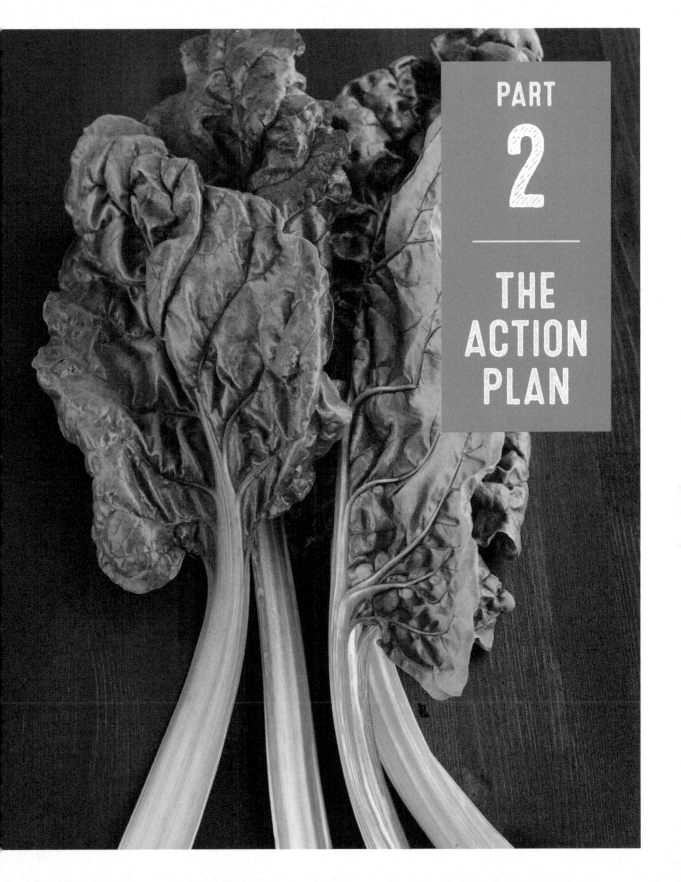

PART

2

THE
ACTION
PLAN

CHAPTER **THREE**

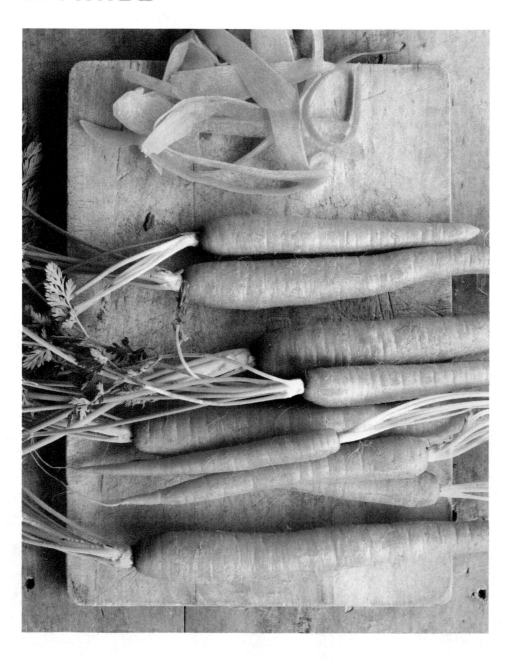

THE ELIMINATION PHASE

Before you start the Autoimmune Paleo Diet, buy a notebook and take a comprehensive head-to-toe inventory of your state of health. Start recording your symptoms, reactions, and emotions at least two weeks before you start the diet, so you have a real sense of what your baseline is. But even doing this just before you start the elimination phase is valuable. This information will be your point of reference for changes that occur during the course of the diet.

The first few days of the elimination plan will be difficult, even if you are enthusiastic about changing your diet. So make sure you go shopping for everything you need and eat simply in the beginning. Try recipes with just a few ingredients and that are within your comfort range for preparation and cooking techniques. All the recipes in this book have preparation times of about 30 minutes or less, so you don't have to live in your kitchen. Make sure you eat at least three meals a day and add a snack if you are hungry, because it is important to start flooding your body with nutrient-dense foods right away to help your gut heal.

The Autoimmune Paleo Diet is not meant to replace any prescriptions and medications that your doctor has recommended for your autoimmune disease, although one of the goals of this healing diet might be to live your life with less medication or even medication-free. Make sure you discuss your diet plan with your doctor before starting, because your medication might have to be adjusted.

30-Day Elimination Meal Plan

There are two ways you can approach the elimination diet. One is to jump right in and the other is to transition slowly. Some people clear out their refrigerator and pantry of excluded foods, go shopping, and start eating Autoimmune Paleo Diet meals immediately. Others want to eliminate each food group individually, one by one, and use up any food that's still in their kitchen until they are completely on the plan. There is no wrong way to begin your journey, so just pick your method and commit; just remember that the 30-day elimination phase does not begin until you've eliminated all of the restricted foods.

The elimination diet is designed to remove all possible gut irritants from your meals to give your body an opportunity to heal. The length of time you follow the plan will depend on your initial physical condition, your autoimmune disease, and the extent of damage that is present in your body. The minimum is 30 days, and the maximum time is not set in stone. Follow the elimination phase of the diet until your symptoms are no longer evident.

You will be cooking the majority (or all) of your meals during the first phase of the diet, and the following meal plan is your map for those first 30 days. The plan includes a variety of proteins, vegetables, and meal choices, each with no more than 20 grams of fructose per day.

You do not have to follow this plan to the letter. It is quite diverse, and you might not have the time to cook every meal. The Autoimmune Paleo Diet is not meant to be a rigid set of diet rules, but rather a flexible template you can use to build your own individual plan. The only rules are to eat nutrient-dense foods every day, eliminate the foods, drinks, and medications listed in chapter 2 (see page 38), follow the lifestyle recommendations, and listen to your body. If you change the meal plans, make sure you also adjust the shopping lists to reflect your changes or you could end up with ingredients that go to waste.

Batch cooking (see page 86) can free up some time by providing Autoimmune Paleo Diet meals that you can pop in the oven from the freezer on busy nights. However, even with batch cooking, be sure to mix up your daily meals; ingredient diversity is the key to getting all the appropriate nutrients in the right amounts to promote healing.

Each week's meal plan has a shopping list associated with it to take the guess work out of trips to the grocery store. These lists probably look long, but in many cases the pantry items, like extra-virgin olive oil and apple cider vinegar, might already be in your cupboards.

Remember to save the bones and carcasses of any proteins you eat to throw in the stockpot for the bone broths. Also, plan ahead and make a batch of pickles a couple of weeks before starting the Autoimmune Paleo Diet (or the week you start), so they are ready to enjoy when you want a crunchy snack. Planning is the key, and in this 30-day plan, we've done all that work for you.

Tips for Success

Be ready for a lifestyle change. The Auto-immune Paleo Diet is not just about the food you eat, although that is obviously the foundation of the diet. You will also have to make changes to your routines. If you are used to heading out after work to enjoy a drink and a plate of pasta with your coworkers, that custom will have to change. Similarly, your grab-and-go cream-filled coffee and donut will also be thrown by the wayside with the Autoimmune Paleo Diet. It is often these changes in your daily routine that can make the Autoimmune Paleo Diet seem too hard. Keep in mind that habits can be replaced, and eventually your green smoothie and bone broth breakfast will also be second nature. Some of the lifestyle modifications you might be making on the Autoimmune Paleo Diet include taking a packed lunch to work or school, cooking in bulk on the weekends, going to bed early, finding time to be physical, and learning to manage your stress in a positive way.

Breakfast will be different. One of the hardest aspects of the Autoimmune Paleo Diet for many people is the fact that they will not be eating traditional breakfast foods. Eggs, toast, cereal, home fries, muffins, croissants with jam, pancakes, and coffee are not on the menu on this diet. Starting the day with this type of food is a habit that is often ingrained from the cradle, so it can be disconcerting to give up the comfort of the familiar. Breakfast can be anything from leftovers to pork sausage with diced sweet potatoes or a nice steak. The idea is to nourish and heal the body, so eat delicious, healthy food and leave the donuts in the box.

Stay the course and ignore negative feedback from others. Support is crucial when you are following the Autoimmune Paleo Diet because it is a difficult diet to undertake and encouragement can be what you need to keep on track. However, if there are people in your life who do not understand what you are trying to achieve, do not give up. In this diet-inundated culture, there is a great deal of faulty information about what is healthy or fattening. Cooking with fat, eating meat, and eliminating grains can seem strange to friends or coworkers, who might feel that your diet is too restrictive. Keep your mind on the goal of alleviating your symptoms and offer to educate naysayers instead of getting defensive or discouraged. Ignorance about the diet or what you are experiencing physically might be the root of a person's negative comments.

30 Days of Meals

You'll find recipes for all the meals in this 30-day plan in part 3. You'll note that desserts are not included in the meal plan; however, everyone needs a treat now and again, especially when the dietary restrictions seem overwhelming. Feel free to pepper your meal plan with desserts from chapter 14.

Day 1
Breakfast: Sweet Broiled Grapefruit
Lunch: Coconut Chicken Fingers
Dinner: Herb-Crusted Salmon
Snack: Naturally Fermented Pickles

Day 2
Breakfast: Breakfast Cookies
Lunch: Grilled Zucchini Salad
Dinner: Simple Vegetable Curry
Snack: Caramel-Coconut Dip

Day 3
Breakfast: Rosy Avocado Smoothie
Lunch: Coconut Seafood Soup
Dinner: Roasted Acorn Squash and
   Brussels Sprouts
Snack: Apple-Bacon Poppers

Day 4
Breakfast: Simple Pork Sausage
Lunch: French Onion Soup
Dinner: Simply Perfect Roast Chicken
Snack: Endive Boats

Day 5
Breakfast: Sweet Potato Bacon
   Hash Browns
Lunch: Simple Borscht
Dinner: Lamb Sliders
Snack: Easy Guacamole

Day 6
Breakfast: Watermelon Smoothie
Lunch: Savory Lamb Stew
Dinner: Shrimp Scampi
Snack: Easy Beef Bone Broth

Day 7
Breakfast: Breakfast Chicken Burgers
Lunch: Fruited Sweet Potato Salad
Dinner: Roasted Spaghetti Squash
   and Kale
Snack: Honey-Thyme Beef Jerky

Day 8
Breakfast: Stuffed Squash
Lunch: Roasted Spaghetti Squash
   and Kale
Dinner: Bacon-Wrapped Venison
Snack: Cut-up vegetables with
   Balsamic Reduction

Day 9

Breakfast: Breakfast "Pizza"
Lunch: Cauliflower-Bacon Soup
Dinner: "Pasta" with Spring Vegetables
Snack: Honeydew Ice Pops

Day 10

Breakfast: Celeriac and Turnip
   Pancakes
Lunch: Jicama-Fennel Salad
Dinner: Tuna Burgers
Snack: Pork and Veggie Meatballs

Day 11

Breakfast: Butternut Squash Porridge
Lunch: Nectarine-Cucumber Salad
Dinner: Lemon-Herb Lamb Cutlets
Snack: Chicken Bone Broth

Day 12

Breakfast: Turkey Breakfast Stir-Fry
Lunch: Fennel-Apple Soup
Dinner: Pear-Stuffed Pork Loin
Snack: Homemade Coconut Yogurt

Day 13

Breakfast: Pumpkin and Ground
   Beef Hash
Lunch: Grapefruit Salad
Dinner: Rosemary Chicken
Snack: Easy Beef Bone Broth

Day 14

Breakfast: Rich Beet Smoothie
Lunch: Roasted Acorn Squash and
   Brussels Sprouts
Dinner: Lime-Infused Poached Salmon
Snack: Turkey Sliders

Day 15

Breakfast: Sweet Potato Bacon
   Hash Browns
Lunch: Grilled Zucchini Salad
Dinner: Stir-Fried Vegetables with
   Cauliflower "Rice"
Snack: Chicken Salad Lettuce Cups

Day 16

Breakfast: Breakfast Cookies
Lunch: Sunny Carrot Soup
Dinner: Coconut Chicken Curry
Snack: Easy Apple Butter

Day 17

Breakfast: Rosy Avocado Smoothie
Lunch: Coconut Chicken Fingers
Dinner: Flank Steak with Lime
   Marinade
Snack: Spiced Peach Spread

Day 18

Breakfast: Stuffed Squash
Lunch: Traditional Coleslaw
Dinner: Lemon Scallops
Snack: Easy Beef Bone Broth

Day 19
Breakfast: Breakfast Chicken Burgers
Lunch: French Onion Soup
Dinner: Lime-Coconut Zucchini
    Noodles with Avocado
Snack: Herbed Mushroom Pâté

Day 20
Breakfast: Rich Beet Smoothie
Lunch: Stuffed Squash
Dinner: Lamb Sliders
Snack: Endive Boats

Day 21
Breakfast: Sweet Potato Bacon
    Hash Browns
Lunch: Radish and Jicama Tabbouleh
Dinner: Cabbage-Turkey Soup
Snack: Easy Guacamole

Day 22
Breakfast: Sweet Potato Breakfast
    Casserole
Lunch: Nectarine-Cucumber Salad
Dinner: Herb-Crusted Salmon
Snack: Roasted Berry Jam

Day 23
Breakfast: Sweet Broiled Grapefruit
Lunch: Roasted Sweet Potato Salad
Dinner: Simply Perfect Roast Chicken
Snack: Pork and Veggie Meatballs

Day 24
Breakfast: Butternut Squash Porridge
Lunch: Coconut Seafood Soup
Dinner: Pot Roast
Snack: Watermelon Granita

Day 25
Breakfast: Simple Pork Sausage
Lunch: Waldorf Salad
Dinner: Simple Vegetable Curry
Snack: Easy Beef Bone Broth

Day 26
Breakfast: Pumpkin and Ground
    Beef Hash
Lunch: Grilled Zucchini Salad
Dinner: Pear-Stuffed Pork Loin
Snack: Honeyed Carrot Mousse

Day 27
Breakfast: Celeriac and Turnip
    Pancakes
Lunch: Fennel-Apple Soup
Dinner: Whole Grilled Trout
    with Herbs
Snack: Easy Apple Butter

Day 28
Breakfast: Breakfast "Pizza"
Lunch: Squash-Pear Soup
Dinner: "Pasta" with Spring Vegetables
Snack: Apple-Bacon Poppers

Day 29
Breakfast: Watermelon Smoothie
Lunch: Stir-Fried Vegetables with
   Cauliflower "Rice"
Dinner: Savory Lamb Stew
Snack: Easy Beef Bone Broth

Day 30
Breakfast: Turkey Breakfast Stir-Fry
Lunch: Jicama-Fennel Salad
Dinner: Traditional Beef Hamburgers
Snack: Strawberry Sorbet

Herbs and Autoimmune Paleo One common concern about Autoimmune Paleo food is that it will be bland and boring. Although some spices and seeds used for flavoring are excluded from this diet, the array of acceptable herbs is considerable. Herbs should always enhance the ingredients you are preparing, not overwhelm them; you can always add more, but you can't take away. Remember to add dried herbs in the early stages of the recipe, usually when you're heating the cooking vessel. Fresh herbs, on the other hand, should be added at the end of the cooking process because herbs lose flavor rapidly if heated longer than about a half an hour.

Weekly Shopping Lists

On these lists, the amounts in parentheses at the end of a line are how much you need for the whole week's worth of recipes. But, for example, you can't just buy five tablespoons of apple cider vinegar, so the shopping list calls for one bottle. Remember, some things on the shopping lists will be the same from week to week. So check your cupboard and refrigerator before you go shopping, and cross off any items that you still have plenty of.

You'll see that this list calls for beef bones and chicken carcasses. For both, make friends with your local butcher shop and someone in the meat department at your local supermarket. Just ask them to save you the beef and chicken bones. They should be very inexpensive. For chicken, you can also use the carcass left over from a roast chicken. As with your meat, look for bones from organic, free-range animals.

Shopping List for Week 1 (Days 1–7)

Fish and Seafood
2 pounds (21 to 25 count) shrimp

3 tilapia fillets

4 (6-ounce) salmon fillets

Meat and Poultry
3 (6-ounce) boneless, skinless
    chicken breasts

1 (4-pound) roasting chicken

1 pound lean ground chicken

2 or 3 chicken carcasses

1½ pounds lamb shoulder

1½ pounds ground lamb

17 slices organic bacon

1 pound ground pork

2 pounds beef, London broil

4 to 6 pounds beef bones (marrow,
    knuckles, ribs, and any other bones)

Fruit
3 pounds apples (9)

5 avocados

2 bananas (1½ cups)

2 red grapefruits

4 lemons

3 limes

1 pint strawberries

1 watermelon (about 2 pounds)

Vegetables and Fungi

1 acorn squash (2 pounds)
6 beets (3 cups)
3 bok choy (1 cup)
1½ pounds Brussels sprouts (6 cups)
1 red cabbage (1½ cups)
27 carrots (5 pounds)
1 celery head (7 stalks)
1 English cucumber
20 to 24 (4-inch) pickling cucumbers
2 endive heads

26 garlic cloves
¾ pound kale (4 cups)
1 lettuce head (4 leaves)
½ pound mushrooms (2½ cups)
6½ pounds sweet onions (20)
1 bunch scallions
1 spaghetti squash (5 pounds)
2 ounces spinach (½ cup)
4 pounds sweet potatoes (12)
2½ pounds zucchini (7)

Herbs

1 bunch fresh basil (9 tablespoons)
1 bunch fresh cilantro (9 tablespoons)
1 (7-inch) piece fresh ginger
   (7 teaspoons)

1 bunch fresh parsley
   (10 tablespoons)
2 bunches fresh thyme
   (5 tablespoons plus 3 sprigs)

Pantry and Refrigerator

1 bottle apple cider vinegar
   (9 tablespoons)
1 jar arrowroot powder (1 tablespoon)
1 box baking soda (1½ teaspoons)
1 bottle gluten-free balsamic vinegar
   (3 tablespoons)
1 jar bay leaves (4 leaves)
1 jar ground cinnamon (5 teaspoons)
1 jar ground cloves (¼ teaspoon)
1 bag coconut flour (10 tablespoons)
3¾ cups shredded unsweetened
   coconut (about 3 pounds)
5 cups unsweetened organic coconut
   milk (if making homemade, buy
   4 cups more shredded unsweetened
   coconut)
1 jar coconut oil (8 tablespoons)

1 package dried cranberries (¾ cup)
5 pitted dates
1 jar garlic powder (1 teaspoon)
1 jar ground ginger (½ teaspoon)
1 jar local organic honey
   (3 tablespoons)
1 bottle maple syrup (¼ cup)
1 bottle extra-virgin olive oil (1¼ cups)
1 jar dried minced onion
   (1 teaspoon)
1 jar sea salt (28 teaspoons)
1 jar dried thyme (1 teaspoon)
1 (5-ounce) BPA-free can
   water-packed tuna
1 jar turmeric (3 teaspoons)

Shopping List for Week 2 (Days 8–14)

Fish and Seafood

4 (6-ounce) salmon fillets

1 (1-pound) sushi-grade tuna fillet

Meat and Poultry

4 (8-ounce) boneless, skinless
    chicken thighs

2 or 3 chicken carcasses

1 (8-ounce) turkey breast

2 pounds ground turkey

12 lamb cutlets (about 1 pound total)

1 (4-pound) boneless pork loin

14 slices organic bacon

1 pound ground pork

3½ pounds lean ground beef

2 to 3 pounds beef bones (marrow,
    knuckles, ribs, and any other bones)

4 (5-ounce) venison steaks

Fruits

1 pound apples (3)

2 red grapefruits

1 honeydew melon (about 1 pound)

11 lemons

2 limes

2 nectarines

2 pears

1 pint raspberries (½ cup)

Vegetables and Fungi

3 acorn squash (6 pounds)

1 pound asparagus (2 cups)

2 beets (1 cup)

1 broccoli head (2 cups florets)

1½ pounds Brussels sprouts (6 cups)

1 butternut squash (3 cups)

8 carrots (1½ pounds)

2 cauliflower heads

1 celeriac root (about 5 cups)

1 celery head (6 stalks)

2 English cucumbers

5 fennel bulbs

17 garlic cloves

1 jicama

¾ pound kale (4 cups)

2 leeks

¾ pound mushrooms (3 cups)

1 red onion (¼ cup)

2 pounds sweet onions (6)

4 parsnips

1 pumpkin (about 2 pounds)

3 cups snap peas

1 spaghetti squash (5 pounds)

1½ pounds spinach (8 cups)

3 turnips (4 cups)

2½ pounds zucchini (7)

Herbs

1 bunch fresh basil (5 tablespoons)

1 bunch fresh cilantro (6 tablespoons)

1 (2-inch) piece fresh ginger
(2 teaspoons)

1 bunch fresh mint (½ cup)

1 bunch fresh oregano (1 tablespoon)

1 bunch fresh parsley (1 cup)

1 bunch fresh rosemary (1 tablespoon)

2 bunches fresh thyme (½ cup)

Pantry and Refrigerator

1 bottle apple cider vinegar
(8 tablespoons)

1 jar arrowroot powder (3 tablespoons)

1 bottle gluten-free balsamic
vinegar (2 cups)

1 jar ground cinnamon (1½ teaspoons)

1 jar ground cloves (¼ teaspoon)

2¼ cups shredded unsweetened
coconut (about 2 pounds)

¼ cup coconut kefir

2 cups unsweetened organic coconut
milk (if making homemade, buy
2 cups more shredded unsweetened
coconut)

1 jar coconut oil (4 tablespoons)

1 bottle coconut water (¼ cup)

1 package dried cranberries (¾ cup)

1 jar ground ginger (1½ teaspoons)

1 jar local organic honey
(1⅓ tablespoons)

¼ cup pastured lard (lard from
pasture-raised beef)

1 bottle extra-virgin olive oil (2 cups)

1 jar dried minced onion (1 teaspoon)

1 package raisins (2 tablespoons)

1 jar sea salt (3¾ teaspoons)

1 jar turmeric (½ teaspoon)

The Cost of Eating Healthfully

The Autoimmune Paleo Diet can be an expensive plan to follow, as is any diet based on meat and organic, high-quality ingredients. Most of the cheaper protein sources, such as eggs and nuts, are eliminated on this diet, as well, so creating a budget-friendly meal plan can be difficult. Here are 10 strategies you can try to make the Autoimmune Paleo Diet more cost-effective.

1 **Shop seasonal and at a farmers' market or directly from the farm.** Seasonal, local fruit and vegetables are not only more delicious and healthier than commercially grown, imported produce, they are also less expensive. When you buy according to the seasons, you will quickly find that farmers have an abundant harvest of ripe produce that they need to sell before it is no longer prime quality. Although getting to the market early in the morning means you'll have the biggest variety, often waiting until the stalls are about to close ensures you can bargain a bit on price, because farmers don't want to haul their goods back home.

2 **Buy bone-in or less expensive cuts of meat.** Prime beef cuts are lovely, but there is a great deal of flavor in less pricy products, such as ground beef and tougher bone-in cuts. The added benefit, beyond saving considerable money, is that you can wrap the bones well and put them in the freezer to be used for bone broth. Also, don't overlook inexpensive organ meats when considering your weekly menu. Liver, heart, and kidneys are very healthy and can be delicious when prepared well. If you can't get used to eating liver by itself, try grinding it up and "hiding" it in ground beef dishes, such as meatloaf and meatballs.

3 **Keep your menu simple.** Although it is nice to experiment with spectacular dishes featuring complex seasonings and unique ingredients, you can save money by sticking to simple, well-prepared meals with a few ingredients, lots of vegetables, and a judicious scattering of herbs. If you want to try out new recipes, do it with dishes that contain familiar ingredients that don't break the bank.

4 **Plan ahead and batch cook.** One of the best strategies to save money is to have a comprehensive meal plan in place before you go shopping. A plan means you can make a shopping list, and you can plan to cook some of your meals in large batches. A list and a plan mean you won't buy items you don't need and you'll waste less food.

5 **Invest in a slow cooker.** It can be the perfect piece of equipment to create tender meat dishes from cuts that are usually tough. You can buy a chuck roast for less money than a better piece of meat, cook it to perfection, and then portion the meat up for convenient ready-made meals.

6 **Buy in bulk.** Buying food in larger quantities tends to be less expensive by the pound than smaller packages. You can divide

up, carefully wrap, and freeze bulk packages of meat or poultry in bags containing just a few servings, or even just one serving. Don't be afraid to take advantage of a sale when you see one, either. For example, if ground beef is a spectacular price, stock up and freeze what you don't need to use at a later date. Items such as coconut oil, olive oil, and spices can be found in bulk stores in large containers. If you don't have a local bulk store, then online shopping can sometimes be a good place to get deals.

7 Buy the whole animal or large parts. Part of what you pay for when buying meat, poultry, and fish is the cost associated with someone cutting it up. A whole fish or chicken might seem more expensive, but after you clean and portion it, the individual parts are much more economical than precut products. Plus you can use the leftover carcasses to make broth.

8 Grow your own produce or pick it yourself. Growing your own food is probably the most cost-efficient way to get quality produce for your table. Planting a big enough garden to make an impact on your grocery bill can be a great deal of work and requires space, but if you have the room, it can be an incredibly rewarding experience. If you cannot have a garden at your home, there are often community sites that offer small plots for gardens. You will need to buy seeds to get started, but after that, there shouldn't be any real expense. If you have no option to grow your own food, consider putting a few pots of fresh herbs on the windowsill. Also, ask at your local farmers' market about farms where you can pick your own apples, vegetables, and other produce. Since you are doing the labor, they will usually be a much cheaper price.

9 Buy high-quality frozen vegetables and fruit. Flash-frozen vegetables lose very few nutrients in the freezing process, and since they are usually frozen when they're ripe, you get quality produce. Frozen vegetables are less expensive than fresh, and you can use exactly what you need and put the rest back in the freezer, which cuts down on waste.

10 Join community-supported agriculture (CSA) programs or farm shares. A CSA is a plan in which you buy a share of a local farmers' produce. After that expense, you will enjoy farm-fresh produce delivered right to your door or to a convenient drop-off location all season long. This arrangement means you get seasonal fruits and vegetables at a much lower price than you would pay in the store. You can even buy a share in a grass-fed cow or pig.

Shopping List for Week 3 (Days 15–21)

Fish and Seafood
2 pounds sea scallops

Meat and Poultry
3 (6-ounce) boneless, skinless
    chicken breasts
4 (8-ounce) boneless, skinless
    chicken breasts
1 pound lean ground chicken

4 to 6 chicken carcasses
1 cup chopped turkey
1½ pounds ground lamb
10 slices organic bacon
1½ pounds flank steak

Fruit
5 pounds apples (15)
6 avocados
2 bananas (1½ cups)
½ cup red grapes
6 lemons
5 limes

1 orange
4 pounds peaches (12)
2 pears
1 pint raspberries (½ cup)
½ pound strawberries (1 cup)

Vegetables
4 acorn squash (8 pounds)
1 pound asparagus (2 cups)
2 beets (1 cup)
1 broccoli head (2 cups florets)
2 green cabbages
1 red cabbage
26 carrots (5 pounds)
1 cauliflower head (4 cups)
1 celery head (11 stalks)
2 English cucumbers
2 endive heads
1 fennel bulb
45 garlic cloves
3 jicamas

1 lettuce head
¼ pound brown button
    mushrooms (1 cup)
¼ pound shitake mushrooms (1 cup)
1 red onion (1 cup)
3½ pounds sweet onions (12 ½)
4 parsnips
9 radishes
1 bunch scallions (4)
1 cup snap peas
3 pounds sweet potatoes (9)
1 winter squash (1 cup)
2½ pounds zucchini (10)

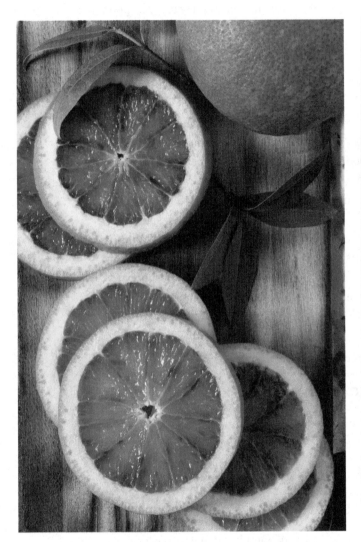

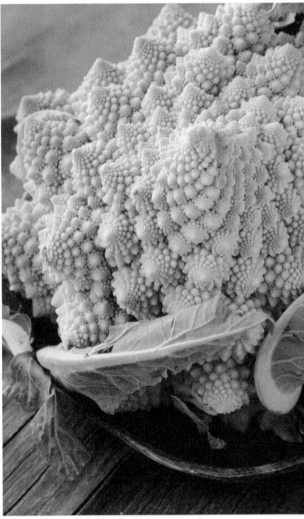

Herbs

1 bunch fresh basil (½ cup)

1 bunch fresh cilantro leaves
(11 tablespoons)

2 (6-inch) pieces fresh ginger
(4 tablespoons)

1 bunch fresh mint (1 tablespoon)

1 bunch fresh parsley (9 tablespoons)

1 bunch fresh tarragon (1 teaspoon)

1 bunch fresh thyme (4 tablespoons)

Pantry and Refrigerator

1 bottle apple cider vinegar
(10 tablespoons)

1 jar arrowroot powder (6 tablespoons)

1 box baking soda (1½ teaspoons)

1 bottle gluten-free balsamic vinegar
(2 tablespoons)

1 jar bay leaves (2 leaves)

1 jar ground cinnamon (8 teaspoons)

1 jar ground cloves (½ teaspoon)

2 cups shredded unsweetened coconut
(about 1½ pounds)

1 jar coconut oil (10 tablespoons)

1 package dried cranberries (1 cup)

6½ cups unsweetened organic coconut
milk (for homemade, buy 4 cups more
shredded unsweetened coconut)

5 pitted dates

1 jar garlic powder (¼ teaspoon)

1 jar ground ginger (1 teaspoon)

1 jar local organic honey (1 tablespoon)

1 bottle extra-virgin olive oil (3 cups)

1 package raisins (4 tablespoons)

1 jar sea salt (2 teaspoons)

1 (5-ounce) BPA-free can
water-packed tuna

1 jar turmeric (2 teaspoons)

Shopping List for Week 4+ (Days 22–30)

Fish and Seafood

10 (21 to 25 count) shrimp

4 (6-ounce) salmon fillets

3 tilapia fillets

1 (2-pound) whole trout

Meat and Poultry

2 (8-ounce) boneless, skinless
chicken breasts

1 (4-pound) roasting chicken

2 or 3 chicken carcasses

2 (8-ounce) turkey breasts

1 pound ground turkey

1½ pounds lamb shoulder

1 (4-pound) boneless pork loin

12 slices organic bacon

2 pounds ground pork

5 pounds lean ground beef

1 (2-pound) chuck roast

Fruits

7½ pounds apples (22)

2 avocados

2 red grapefruits

1 cup green grapes

11 lemons

2 nectarines

4 pears

½ pound raspberries

1 pound fresh strawberries

2 cups frozen strawberries

1 watermelon (about 2 pounds)

Vegetables and Fungi

1 pound asparagus (2 cups)

3 bok choy (1 cup)

2 broccoli heads (4 cups florets)

1 butternut squash (3 cups)

1 red cabbage (½ cup)

24 carrots (4½ pounds)

1 celeriac root (about 5 cups)

1 celery head (16 stalks)

4 English cucumbers

4 fennel bulbs

30 garlic cloves

1 jicama

1 lettuce head (4 leaves)

1 pound mushrooms (5½ cups)

1 red onion

3½ pounds sweet onions (10)

2 parsnips

1 pumpkin (about 2 pounds)

5 cups snap peas

1 pound spinach (5½ cups)

5½ pounds sweet potatoes (16)

3 turnips (4 cups)

1 winter squash (about 3 pounds)

7 pounds zucchini (14)

Herbs

1 bunch fresh basil (13 tablespoons)

1 bunch fresh cilantro (4 tablespoons)

1 (8-inch) piece fresh ginger
   (8 teaspoons)

1 bunch fresh mint (½ cup plus
   6 leaves)

1 bunch fresh oregano (1 tablespoon)

1 bunch fresh parsley (9 tablespoons)

2 bunches fresh thyme
   (13½ teaspoons plus 11 sprigs)

Pantry and Refrigerator

1 bottle apple cider vinegar (¾ cup)

1 jar arrowroot powder (2 tablespoons)

1 bottle gluten-free balsamic vinegar
   (2 tablespoons)

1 jar ground cinnamon (5¼ teaspoons)

1 jar ground cloves (1¼ teaspoons)

¼ cup shredded, unsweetened
   coconut (¼ pound)

1 small bag coconut flour
   (2 teaspoons)

4 cups unsweetened organic coconut milk
(for homemade, buy 2 cups shredded
unsweetened coconut)

1 jar coconut oil (5 tablespoons)

1 package dried cranberries (¼ cup)

4 tablespoons unflavored gelatin

1 jar ground ginger (2 teaspoons)

1 jar local organic honey
(2 tablespoons)

¼ cup pastured lard

1 bottle extra-virgin olive oil (1½ cups)

1 jar dried minced onion (1 teaspoon)

1 jar sea salt (5¼ teaspoons)

1 jar turmeric (2½ teaspoons)

Batch Cooking

Batch cooking is when you cook more than one meal at a time or components of several meals to freeze or store in the refrigerator for convenient use later in the week or month. You don't have to commit to batch cooking an entire week of food, but even doubling a favorite recipe and freezing the extra dish can put you ahead. Here are some tips to successfully batch cook for your Autoimmune Paleo Diet journey.

- Make sure you have a food plan that uses similar ingredients, so you can cut down on cost and preparation time. Shop for everything at once, and take advantage of any large cuts of meat or bulk vegetables for your batch dishes.

- Prepare and refrigerate large batches of staple items and recipe components such as roast chicken, browned ground beef, and chopped vegetables to use later in the week.

- Use a food processor whenever possible to chop your vegetables in bulk for all your recipes at once. Chopping eight or nine onions can be daunting if you have only a knife and a cutting board.

- When doubling a recipe, make sure you taste it before simply doubling the seasonings. Doubling some spices can over-season a dish. Add just a little more than is called for in a single batch, then taste and add more if necessary.

- Undercook your vegetables slightly if you are freezing them, because you will be reheating the dish. Do not freeze cabbage, celery, or parsley, because they can get very mushy. If your recipe calls for these ingredients, lightly sauté them and then add them when you reheat the dish.

- Separate your dishes into usable portions before you freeze it, such as 1-cup containers of chicken bone broth, so that you can take out what you need without wasting the rest.

- Make sure your food is cooled thoroughly to room temperature before you put a lid on your containers or seal your freezer bags. Freeze your cooled dishes immediately so that they are safe, without any chance of bacterial growth. Remove as much air as possible from freezer bags to prevent freezer burn.

- Have all the tools necessary on hand when you batch cook, such as the correct size and number of containers, freezer bags, and labels. Label your containers with what's inside, the date you made it, and any reheating directions you might need.

How to Track Your Symptoms in the Elimination Phase

Each person's autoimmune journey will be unique to them, so your reaction to the elimination phase of the diet will also be unique. It is impossible to predict how long you will have to follow the elimination portion of the diet, so it's important to track your physical reactions to pinpoint when you can start reintroducing foods. Ideally, you should record all your symptoms in detail at least two weeks before starting the Autoimmune Paleo Diet, so that you have a baseline from which to compare. Write down what you eat, when you eat it, immediate responses (if there are any), and any symptoms that worsen or change after a meal. A list of chronic symptoms is also valuable.

If you follow the plan for several months and see no improvement or very little, it can be beneficial to discuss the situation with your doctor to pinpoint what might be stalling your progress. You might need supplements or tests to determine the best ways to modify your approach.

It is also valuable to look very closely at how well you are complying with the food limits and lifestyle changes. If you include the occasional handful of nuts several times a week or have been burning the midnight oil for work, then you might have to adhere more closely to the plan to see results. Here are some questions to ask yourself if you are not seeing improvements in your symptoms.

- Am I following the Autoimmune Paleo Diet strictly?

- Am I eating a wide enough variety of ingredients?

- Am I including healing foods such as bone broth, offal, and probiotic foods?

- Am I drinking enough water—at least eight glasses a day and not with my meals? Staying hydrated is important, so you should drink 64 ounces of water per day. However, don't drink your water during meals, because this will dilute the enzymes in your mouth and alter the pH in your saliva, which will make it more difficult to digest carbohydrates, starches, and sugars.

- Do I eat mindfully, with no distractions, and chew my food thoroughly?

- Do I allow time after eating and before starting an activity, so my body can digest the food?

- Am I taking the supplements and medications required to support my digestive system, address micronutrient deficiencies, and support gut health?

- Am I getting eight to ten hours of sleep a night?
- Am I managing my stress?
- Am I spending time outside in the sunshine and using dim lights in my home at night?
- Do I get moderate exercise regularly?
- Are my blood sugar levels in a healthy range?
- Have I been tested for food allergies, heavy metal poisoning, hormone imbalance, thyroid function, and small intestinal bacterial over-growth (SIBO)?
- Have I considered cutting down on or stopping medications, under the supervision of a doctor, that undermine the healing process?
- Do I laugh and spend quality time with loved ones every day?

CHAPTER FOUR

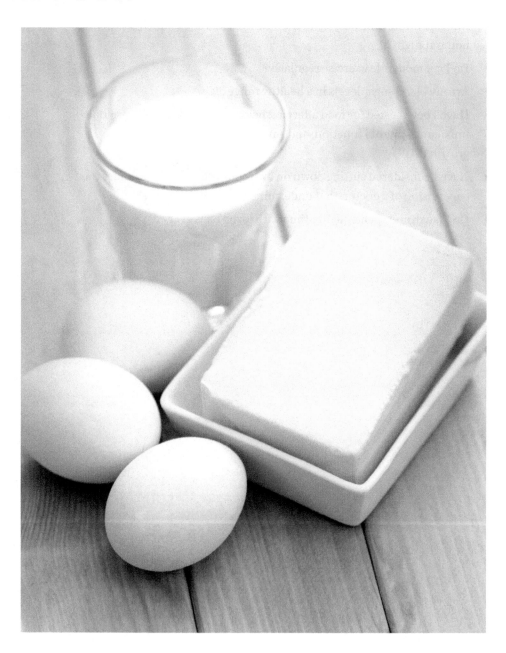

THE REINTRODUCTION PHASE

Successfully reintroducing foods can be a huge boost to morale and make you feel excited about the prospect of enjoying what might have been a favorite food. However, it is very important not to rush this process, because the longer you allow your body to heal, the better the chance of success during the reintroductions.

Wait a minimum of 30 days with no cheating, and maintain the Autoimmune Paleo Diet for three to six months, if you can stick with the elimination phase that long. You should not attempt to reintroduce any food until all your symptoms have improved considerably or subsided completely. You should also be following the lifestyle recommendations, because sleep, stress, and the amount of exercise you do can have a profound effect on your symptoms. You don't want to inadvertently sabotage yourself during the reintroduction process. It would be awful to attribute a reaction to a challenge food when it is actually because you overdid your workout at the gym.

You also have to be emotionally and mentally prepared for the possibility that you might not be able to eat certain foods. Don't let this prospect scare you, because that fear response can exacerbate your symptoms. Approach the reintroduction phase as an experiment—which it is!—and don't fret. Even if you can't tolerate a challenge food now, you can always try it again after six months. Food intolerances sometimes fade or change.

How to Reintroduce Foods

In the reintroduction phase, it can take a substantial amount of time to work through the list of eliminated foods. You have to reintroduce them one by one, so you know exactly how you react to that and only that food. But in the end you will know exactly which foods can be included in your diet and which to avoid. The reintroduction process is simple, but you need to follow it strictly.

1. Pick just one challenge food.

2. Start with small amounts of the food. Try ½ teaspoon and wait 15 to 30 minutes to see if you have a reaction. If you have no reaction, try 1 teaspoon of the food and wait 15 minutes to gauge your reaction. If you have no reaction, then eat 1½ teaspoons of the food and wait two to three hours to see if you have any reaction. If you have a reaction at any point in this process, stop eating the food.

3. If eating small amounts of the challenge food causes no reaction, the next day eat a normal portion of the challenge food.

4. Monitor your body for three days after the normal portion (don't eat any more of the food for those three days). Reactions are not always immediate, and it can take up to three days for symptoms to manifest. Look for changes such as sleep disruption, rashes, mental fog, respiratory problems, joint pain, inflammation, exhaustion, or digestive issues. If you have any of these problems, then you are intolerant and should not eat the challenge food. If you have a reaction, make sure your symptoms completely subside before trying the next challenge food. It may take a few days.

5. If after three days you have no problems, try a greater exposure to the food by eating a little every day for a week. Sometimes reactions are more subtle than acute, and you only notice a problem when you eat the

---

Autoimmune Paleo and Eating Out Going out for dinner is more than just a culinary experience; it is how we interact with friends and family—even how we do business. Following the Autoimmune Paleo diet does not mean you cannot enjoy a good meal out on the town. Of course, a bit of research will be required to find a restaurant that's able to meet your needs. Call ahead to see how the chef handles specific restrictions—some gleefully accept the challenge while others stick to a set menu. Keep your choices simple and make reservations ahead of time so that the kitchen can take precautions to avoid cross contamination in your dish.

---

food for a week. If you have no reaction during this week-long exposure, the food is safe to add back to your diet, and you can go on to the next challenge food.

Which Foods to Reintroduce First

In the reintroduction phase, it's a good idea to introduce foods first that are less likely to cause reactions. This increases the chances of success and won't leave you with a serious flare-up because you tried potatoes or tomatoes first. The order suggested here is by no means the only possible one. And if you really miss a particular food, like coffee or almonds, then try that first. Your food intolerances are unique to you, so there is no way to predict which foods you will tolerate and which ones will cause reactions.

Based on the likelihood of developing a reaction, reintroduce these foods one at a time, in this order.

- Egg yolks (from free-range, soy-free chickens)
- Raw fresh snap peas or green beans
- Fruit-based spices
- Seed-based spices
- Seed oils
- Nut oils
- Ghee (from grass-fed cows)
- Seeds (and seed butters, seed flours, raw seeds, and toasted seeds)
- Nuts (and nut butters, nut flours, raw nuts, and toasted nuts—except cashews and pistachios)
- Cocoa (in homemade chocolate, if possible, because commercial chocolate has fillers that include dairy, gluten, and sugar)
- Egg whites (from free-range, soy-free chickens)
- Butter (from grass-fed cows)
- Alcohol (in very small quantities)
- Cashews and pistachios (they are members of the poison ivy family and should be reintroduced later than the other nuts)
- Coffee (brew your own at home)

- Cream (from grass-fed cows)
- Fermented dairy products (such as yogurt)
- Eggplants
- Sweet bell peppers
- Paprika
- Milk (from grass-fed cows)
- Cheese (from grass-fed cows)
- Chili peppers
- Tomatoes
- Potatoes
- Nightshade spices
- Alcohol (in larger quantities)

How to Track Your Symptoms in the Reintroduction Phase

During the reintroduction phase it is important to track what you eat and your symptoms, so you have an accurate record of what goes on in your body. Write everything down, both positive and negative, to get a clear idea about how foods affect your body. Keep track of other aspects of your life, too, so that a big stressful project at work doesn't cause you to discount a challenge food.

Meditation as a Tool   Stress can have a negative effect on the autoimmune response, so learning to manage stress can help control flares and improve your health. Avoiding stress completely is unrealistic, but meditation can be a powerful tool to managing your stress levels. There are many methods and types of meditation available through yoga classes, community centers, and smartphone apps. Meditation is not limited to the stereotypical lotus position; you can walk, listen to music, swim, cycle, or do any other activity that leaves your mind free. You just need to find an environment that allows you to center yourself and let go of everything but the mindfulness of the moment. Meditation is an individual process and after learning the basic skills from a teacher, video, or book, you can adapt the practice for your own needs.

Who's Eating Paleo?

More and more celebrities and athletes are adopting a Paleo diet—some to help them deal with health issues and others because they like the way the diet makes them look and feel. So who's eating Paleo?

Jack Osbourne, son of Sharon and Ozzy Osbourne, has multiple sclerosis. "At its core, I look at MS as inflammation, so I try and eliminate foods that cause inflammation: dairy, gluten, and grains," Osbourne told ABC News.

Jessica Biel said in an interview with CrossFit Zone that her Paleo diet "just leans you down and slims you up and takes that little layer of fat, skin, and water weight right off your body."

Miley Cyrus has gluten and lactose allergies. "Everyone should try no gluten for a week!" she told *US Weekly*. "The change in your skin, physical, and mental health is amazing. You won't go back!"

Among athletes, LA Clippers star Grant Hill says his Paleo lifestyle is what has kept him fit through his 19 years in the NBA. "I think I'll wear out mentally before I will physically," he told *Paleo Lifestyle Magazine*.

Things to track include:

- Sleep habits and how you feel when you wake up (rested, troubled, or fatigued upon waking)
- Energy levels
- Digestion
- Skin
- Emotions
- Pain and where (rated on a 0 to 10 scale)
- Any autoimmune disease symptoms and any changes
- Any other changes in your routine
- The challenge food you are working on

Troubleshooting

During the reintroduction process, you might find yourself dealing with a range of emotions. It is important to accept and diffuse these emotions because they can act as stressors on your body. Use stress management and relaxation techniques to deal with your emotions in a healthy way, such as yoga, a hug from a friend, a massage, meditation, music, exercise, or deep-breathing exercises.

If a challenge food causes a flare-up, you will have to deal with the physical and emotional response in your body. It is best to look at the reaction as a furthering of your knowledge about your body. You are now armed with information that allows you to avoid future damage due to that challenge food. If you stop eating the food, your body will heal again.

Here are some strategies you can use to get through a flare-up during the reintroduction process.

- Take care of yourself and ask for help.

- Some autoimmune diseases are characterized by intense pain during flare-ups, and if this is the case for you, relieve the pain with medication if you have to. Pain is an extreme stressor, and it is unhealthy to suffer through it.

- Get quality sleep. The body heals during sleep, and flare-ups can be utterly exhausting. Go to bed early, nap, and relax until you feel better.

- Eat nutrient-dense foods and healing foods such as bone broth and seafood. Have a loved one make a soothing, nutritious pot of soup to help you through the flare-up.

- Take a relaxing, detoxifying bath with Epsom salts or herbs.

- Get outside and soak up some sun and vitamin D.

- Practice positive reinforcement thinking by visualizing yourself healthy and flare-up free, rather than obsessing about your symptoms.

- Document anything that relieves the flare-up faster or has no effect, so you have a strategy for another incident.

- Cuddle up and hug someone you love (a person or a pet) because it feels lovely and releases a hormone called oxytocin that calms the body and elevates mood.

PART 3

THE RECIPES

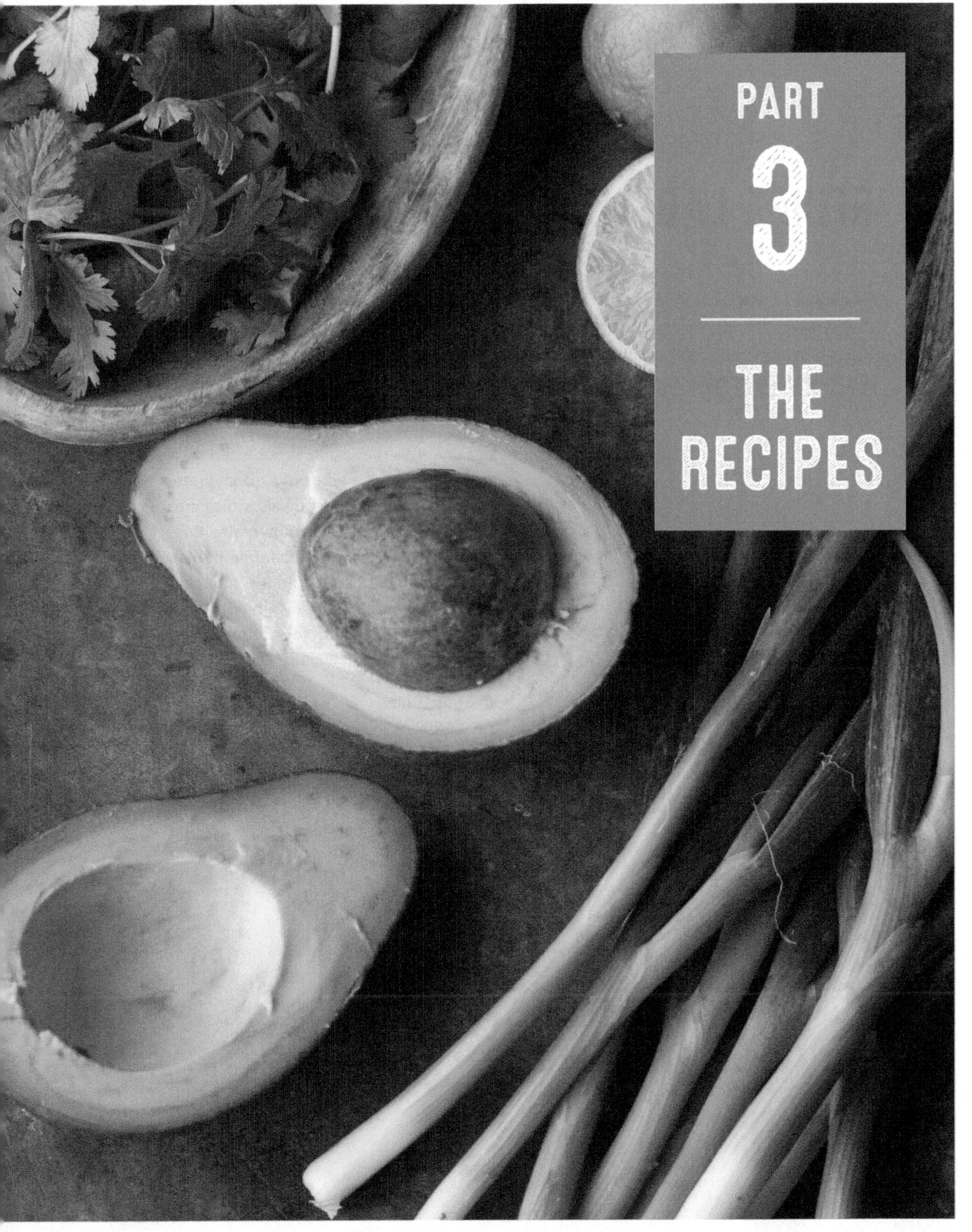

RECIPE LABELS

Throughout the recipes in the following chapters, you'll find a number of helpful labels that highlight certain attributes. Here's what each label means.

FODMAP-FREE

This may be a diet you are unfamiliar with if you do not suffer from Crohn's disease, irritable bowel syndrome, or colitis. It is designed to provide relief from the unpleasant symptoms associated with these conditions, such as abdominal pain, bloating, bowel changes, and gas. This diet came about when studies showed that some types of carbohydrates caused irritation in the bowels, which creates these symptoms. The carbohydrates that affect the bowels are called fermentable oligosaccharides, disaccharides, monosaccharides, and polyols, known by the acronym FODMAP. The range of foods that are not allowed on this diet include:

- Some fruits
- Some vegetables, including all alliums (such as onions, garlic, and chives)
- Grains and cereals
- Some nuts
- Sugars and other sweeteners
- Prebiotic foods
- Some alcohols
- Dairy foods

MAKE AHEAD

Recipes that hold well in the fridge or freezer and can be reheated with no loss of texture or flavor. These are also dishes that could require marinating time or need to sit for the flavors to mature. Make ahead recipes are good choices if you want to cook several meals on the weekend and serve them later in the week to save time.

QUICK+EASY

You will be able to finish the preparation and cooking of these recipes in 30 minutes or less. Some of the recipes may require freezing or marinating but the active work or cooking is under that time frame.

KIDS' FAVORITE

Recipes that are appealing to kids, even picky eaters. These dishes can be fun, colorful, sweeter, or less spicy or are very close to traditional family favorite recipes.

GOOD FOR BATCHES

Batch cooking is when you cook more than one meal at a time or components of several meals to freeze or store in the refrigerator for convenient use later in the week or month. These recipes can also be doubled for times you want leftovers or are feeding a large group of people.

CHAPTER FIVE

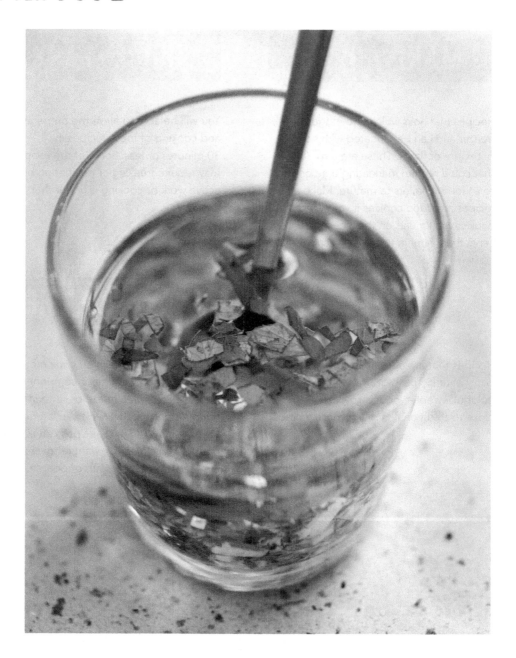

SAUCES AND MARINADES

STEAK AND POULTRY SPICE RUB

MAKE AHEAD | QUICK+EASY | GOOD FOR BATCHES

▶ Makes 1 cup (1 tablespoon per serving)

▶ Prep time: 5 minutes

Well-seasoned food is a joy to create and consume. This versatile spice rub has a rich, garlicky undertone accented with a mix of herbs that impart a Mediterranean flavor. The blend of tastes works beautifully with most kinds of meat, and with chicken, too. Experiment with your quail, bison, and lamb next time you are roasting or barbecuing.

¼ cup garlic powder

2 tablespoons dried minced onion

2 tablespoons dried oregano

2 tablespoons dried thyme

1 tablespoon sea salt

½ teaspoon ground ginger

½ teaspoon dried marjoram

1. Stir the garlic, onion, oregano, thyme, salt, ginger, and marjoram in a small bowl until well combined.

2. Transfer the spice mixture to a sealed container, and store it in a cool dark place for up to 2 months.

SAUCES AND MARINADES

PER SERVING
CALORIES: 11
TOTAL FAT: 0 G
SODIUM: 352 MG
CARBS: 2 G
SUGAR: 1 G
PROTEIN: 1 G

BALSAMIC REDUCTION

FODMAP-FREE | MAKE AHEAD | GOOD FOR BATCHES

- ▸ Makes 1 cup (1 tablespoon per serving)
- ▸ Prep time: 0 minutes ▸ Cook time: 15 to 20 minutes

If you have never tried a drizzle of balsamic reduction on a salad, a piece of meat, or fruit such as peaches or strawberries, you are in for a treat. It's important to buy a good-quality aged balsamic vinegar for this recipe to produce the perfect sweet richness. Make sure you use a nonreactive pot to create the reduction, and turn the fan on above your stove to suck up the strong scent of cooking vinegar.

2 cups gluten-free balsamic vinegar

1. Pour the vinegar in a nonreactive, medium saucepan, and place the pan over medium-high heat.

2. Bring the vinegar to a boil and reduce the heat to low.

3. Simmer the vinegar until it thickens, reduces, and coats the back of a spoon, 15 to 20 minutes. Watch it carefully in the last 5 minutes so it doesn't burn.

4. Let the reduction cool for about 20 minutes.

5. Transfer the reduction to a sealed container and allow it to cool completely before storing it in the refrigerator for up to 1 month.

6. If the reduction becomes too thick to drizzle, add a little water to thin it out to the right consistency.

SAUCES AND MARINADES

PER SERVING
CALORIES: 6
TOTAL FAT: 0 G
SODIUM: 2 MG
CARBS: 0 G
SUGAR: 0 G
PROTEIN: 0 G

GARLIC-CITRUS MARINADE

MAKE AHEAD | QUICK+EASY | GOOD FOR BATCHES

- ▸ Makes about 2 cups (2 tablespoons per serving)
- ▸ Prep time: 15 minutes

Using marinades is an easy way to enhance the flavor of meats, seafood, poultry, and vegetables. This recipe uses acid from the citrus fruits as a base, so only marinate your food about 1 to 2 hours maximum to avoid having a tough finished dish. If you are marinating shrimp, add 1 teaspoon of ginger to create a delightful Asian taste. Lemons and limes are very high in vitamin C, which is a very powerful antioxidant. Antioxidants neutralize free radicals in the body, which helps reduce inflammation and boost the immune system. Free radicals are oxygen or nitrogen molecules that do not have electrons in complete sets, so they damage the body by taking electrons from surrounding cells to complete the electron set.

1 cup extra-virgin olive oil

Juice and zest of 1 lemon

Juice and zest of 1 lime

Juice and zest of ½ orange

2 teaspoons minced garlic

1 teaspoon dried thyme or 1 tablespoon chopped fresh thyme

½ teaspoon sea salt

1. Place the olive oil, lemon juice and zest, lime juice and zest, orange juice and zest, garlic, thyme, and salt in a small jar, seal it, and shake it until well combined.

2. Store the marinade in the jar in the refrigerator for up to 1 week.

PER SERVING
CALORIES: 113
TOTAL FAT: 13 G
SODIUM: 59 MG
CARBS: 1 G
SUGAR: 0 G
PROTEIN: 0 G

HERBED GREEK DRESSING

MAKE AHEAD | *KIDS' FAVORITE* | *QUICK+EASY* | GOOD FOR BATCHES

- ▶ Makes 1 cup (1 tablespoon per serving)
- ▶ Prep time: 4 minutes

Greek cuisine highlights fresh vegetables, meats, and seafood found in the region. The herbs and spices used in Greek recipes enhance rather than mask the flavors of the other ingredients. This dressing uses oregano, the most widely used herb in Greek cuisine, which combines beautifully with the subtle sweet acid of the balsamic vinegar.

¾ cup extra-virgin olive oil
¼ cup gluten-free balsamic vinegar
2 tablespoons chopped fresh oregano or 2 teaspoons dried oregano
1 tablespoon minced garlic
¼ teaspoon sea salt

1. Whisk the olive oil and vinegar in a small bowl until emulsified, about 3 minutes.

2. Whisk in the oregano, garlic, and salt until well combined, about 1 minute.

3. Transfer the dressing to a sealed container, and store it in the refrigerator for up to 1 week. Shake the dressing before using it.

SAUCES AND MARINADES

PER SERVING
CALORIES: 83
TOTAL FAT: 9 G
SODIUM: 31 MG
CARBS: 0 G
SUGAR: 0 G
PROTEIN: 0 G

LEMON DRESSING

MAKE AHEAD | QUICK+EASY | GOOD FOR BATCHES

▶ Makes about 2 cups (2 tablespoons per serving)

▶ Prep time: 5 minutes

Lemon is one of the most popular flavors in the world, across many different cultures and cuisines. The tartness of the fruit combines well with almost any other ingredient, including the sublime pairing with honey in this dressing. Citrus is an allowed food on the Autoimmune Paleo Diet list, but people can have individual food allergies to this family of fruit. If you are sensitive to citrus, remove the lemon juice and increase the vinegar in the recipe to 1/2 cup.

SAUCES AND MARINADES

PER SERVING
CALORIES: 126
TOTAL FAT: 13 G
SODIUM: 17 MG
CARBS: 5 G
SUGAR: 5 G
PROTEIN: 0 G

1 cup extra-virgin olive oil

1/2 cup freshly squeezed lemon juice

1/4 cup honey

2 tablespoons apple cider vinegar

1 teaspoon chopped fresh basil

Pinch sea salt

1. Whisk the olive oil, lemon juice, honey, vinegar, thyme, and salt in a small bowl until well combined.

2. Transfer the dressing to a sealed container and store it in the refrigerator for up to 2 weeks.

3. Take the dressing out about 15 minutes before you want to use it and shake it well before pouring it on your salad.

TOMATO-FREE "MARINARA" SAUCE

- ▸ Makes 5 to 6 cups (1 cup per serving)
- ▸ Prep time: 15 minutes ▸ Cook time: 30 minutes

Marinara sauce is a traditional Italian staple made from tomatoes, onion, garlic, and herbs. While this recipe is obviously not a tomato sauce, it does have all the other ingredients and can be used in the same way in your recipes. You will find a complexity of flavor in this sauce due to the multitude of vegetables and a satisfying natural sweetness that might make you forget all your experiences with tomato-based marinara sauces. Bellissimo!

2 cups peeled, cubed butternut squash

1 cup peeled, chopped sweet potato

3 carrots, peeled and chopped

2 beets, peeled and quartered

2 celery stalks, sliced

½ sweet onion, chopped

4 teaspoons minced garlic

1 tablespoon extra-virgin olive oil

½ cup water, or as needed

2 tablespoons fresh chopped parsley

1 tablespoon fresh chopped basil or 1 teaspoon dried basil

1 tablespoon fresh chopped oregano or 1 teaspoon dried oregano

¼ teaspoon sea salt

SAUCES AND MARINADES

PER SERVING

CALORIES: 83

TOTAL FAT: 3 G

SODIUM: 131 MG

CARBS: 24 G

SUGAR: 9 G

PROTEIN: 2 G

1. Place the squash, sweet potato, carrots, beets, and celery in a large saucepan and cover them with about 2 inches of water.

2. Place the saucepan on medium-high heat and bring to a boil.

3. Reduce the heat to low and simmer the vegetables until they are fork tender, about 20 minutes.

4. Drain and transfer the vegetables to a food processor.

5. While the vegetables are cooking, sauté the onion and garlic in a small skillet in the olive oil until tender, about 3 minutes. ▸

Tomato-Free "Marinara" Sauce *continued*

6. Add the onion and garlic to the food processor with the cooked vegetables and pulse until the sauce is smooth.

7. Add the water, as needed, to create a thick, pourable sauce.

8. Pour the sauce back into the saucepan and add the parsley, basil, oregano, and salt.

9. Simmer the sauce for about 5 minutes to combine the flavors.

10. Remove the saucepan from the heat and let the sauce cool for 15 minutes.

11. Transfer the sauce to a sealed container and store it in the refrigerator for up to 4 days.

12. Reheat and serve the sauce over meat, poultry, fish, vegetables, or zucchini noodles.

SAUCES AND
MARINADES

SWEET BARBECUE SAUCE

MAKE AHEAD | KIDS' FAVORITE | QUICK+EASY | GOOD FOR BATCHES

- ▸ Makes 2 cups (2 tablespoons per serving)
- ▸ Prep time: 15 minutes ▸ Cook time: 20 minutes

There are serious competitions for the best barbecue sauce, and people spend hours, days, and even years perfecting their version of this humble condiment. This recipe takes little more than half an hour to create a winning combination that is sweet, tart, and smoky, with a delightful touch of heat. Although coconut oil is an acceptable option to use in this recipe, try making at least one batch with reserved bacon fat, because that flavor component elevates the sauce to sublime. To save money when cherries are out of season, try using flash frozen, no-sugar-added cherries. Simply thaw them out in the quantity you need and follow the recipe as if you were using fresh fruit.

1 tablespoon bacon fat or coconut oil
1 sweet onion, chopped
1 teaspoon minced garlic
1 cup pitted black cherries
½ cup peeled and chopped carrot
4 tablespoons maple syrup
2 tablespoons apple cider vinegar
1 teaspoon ground ginger
¼ teaspoon smoked sea salt
Pinch ground cloves

SAUCES AND
MARINADES

PER SERVING
CALORIES: 30
TOTAL FAT: 1 G
SODIUM: 46 MG
CARBS: 6 G
SUGAR: 5 G
PROTEIN: 0 G

1. Place the bacon fat in a large saucepan over medium-high heat and sauté the onion and garlic until translucent, about 3 minutes.

2. Add the cherries, carrot, maple syrup, and vinegar, and stir to combine.

3. Cook the mixture, crushing the cherries against the sides of the saucepan, until the liquid simmers, about 3 minutes.

4. Reduce the heat and simmer the sauce, stirring frequently, until the carrots are tender, about 10 minutes. ▸

Sweet Barbecue Sauce *continued*

5. Add the ginger, salt, and cloves, and simmer the sauce for 4 more minutes.

6. Transfer the mixture to a blender and blend until it is smooth, about 1 minute.

7. Transfer the sauce to a container and cool it in the refrigerator before sealing the container. Store the sauce in the sealed container in the refrigerator for up to 1 week.

SAUCES AND
MARINADES

ITALIAN MARINADE

- ▸ Makes 3 cups
- ▸ Prep time: 10 minutes

This marinade is one of the most versatile you will have in your culinary repertoire. You can use it with seafood, fish, poultry, and red meat before either baking or grilling your proteins. This flavorful mixture can also shine as a delicious dressing for salads, especially spinach or romaine lettuces. If you do not have the exact combination of herbs required in the ingredients, you can easily swap them around with whatever is in your fridge or garden.

1½ cups olive oil

¼ cup wine vinegar

¼ cup freshly squeezed lemon juice

¼ cup minced sweet onion

¼ cup chopped fresh flat leaf parsley

¼ cup chopped fresh basil

1 tablespoon chopped fresh oregano

1 tablespoon chopped fresh thyme

1 tablespoon minced fresh garlic

⅛ teaspoon sea salt

SAUCES AND MARINADES

PER SERVING

CALORIES: 74

TOTAL FAT: 8G

SODIUM: 10MG

CARBS: 1G

SUGAR: 0G

PROTEIN: 0G

1. Whisk together the olive oil, vinegar, and lemon juice until well blended.

2. Add the onion, parsley, basil, oregano, thyme, garlic, and sea salt.

3. Whisk until well combined and transfer the marinade to a sealed container.

4. Store in the fridge for up to 1 week.

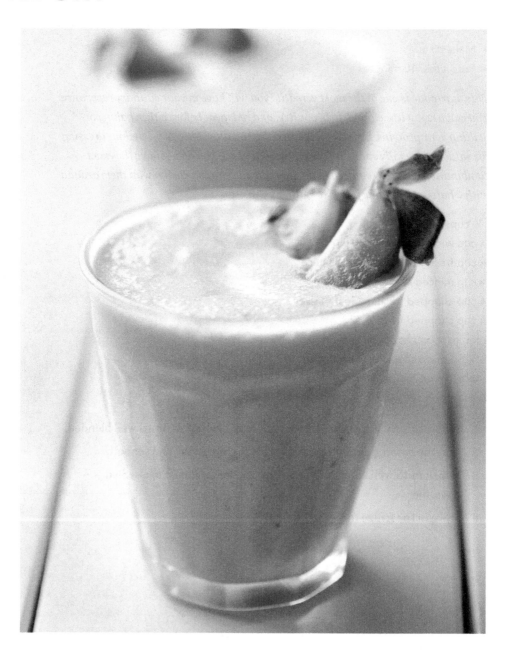

BREAKFASTS

ROSY AVOCADO SMOOTHIE

FODMAP-FREE | KIDS' FAVORITE | QUICK+EASY

▸ Serves 2

▸ Prep time: 10 minutes

The rosiness in this pale, pretty smoothie comes from the strawberries. Berries of any type are a wonderful choice on the Autoimmune Paleo Diet because they are low in sugar and very high in vitamins, minerals, and disease-fighting antioxidants. If you want a cold treat, try substituting frozen organic strawberries for the fresh berries in this recipe.

2 cups unsweetened organic coconut milk (for homemade, see page 258)

1 avocado, peeled, pitted, and cut into quarters

1 cup strawberries

¼ teaspoon ground cinnamon

1. Add the coconut milk and avocado to a blender and purée until smooth.

2. Add the strawberries and cinnamon and pulse until the smoothie is thick and the desired texture.

3. Pour the smoothie into 2 glasses and serve.

BREAKFASTS

PER SERVING

CALORIES: 274

TOTAL FAT: 24 G

SODIUM: 22 MG

CARBS: 16 G

SUGAR: 5 G

PROTEIN: 2 G

WATERMELON SMOOTHIE

KIDS' FAVORITE | QUICK+EASY

▸ Serves 2
▸ Prep time: 15 minutes

Red cabbage is the surprise ingredient in this smoothie, but don't worry; its pungent taste is lost in the sweet, refreshing presence of the watermelon. Cabbage is a cruciferous vegetable, which means it has lots of healthy fiber and important cancer-fighting properties. Cruciferous vegetables also have goitrogenic properties that can interfere with iodine uptake, which affects how the thyroid functions. The amount of cabbage in this smoothie is very small, so it should not have a detrimental effect. However, if you have a severe iodine deficiency, do not eat large quantities of these vegetables until the condition is addressed.

1 cup sliced English cucumber
½ cup shredded red cabbage
2 cups diced watermelon
1 cup ice

1. Add the cucumber and cabbage to a blender and pulse until they are chopped into very small pieces, about 2 minutes.

2. Add the watermelon and pulse until the smoothie is well combined, about 1 minute.

3. Add the ice and blend until the smoothie is thick and smooth. If the drink is too thick, add a little water until you have the right consistency.

4. Pour the smoothie into 2 glasses and serve.

PER SERVING
CALORIES: 58
TOTAL FAT: 0 G
SODIUM: 6 MG
CARBS: 14 G
SUGAR: 10 G
PROTEIN: 2 G

RICH BEET SMOOTHIE

FODMAP-FREE | QUICK+EASY

- ▶ Serves 2
- ▶ Prep time: 10 minutes

Roasting beets intensifies their sweetness and adds a lovely smoky undertone. This enhanced richness combines with tart raspberries to create a smoothie that might become your favorite breakfast treat. Although beets are available year-round, the best young beets are found from June to October.

1 cup diced roasted beets

1 cup unsweetened organic coconut milk (for homemade, see page 258)

1 cup diced fennel bulb

½ cup raspberries

1 cup ice

1. Place the beets, coconut milk, fennel, and raspberries in a blender and pulse until smooth, about 3 minutes.

2. Add the ice and blend until the smoothie is thick and smooth, about 1 minute. If the drink is too thick, add a little water until you have the right consistency.

3. Pour the smoothie into 2 glasses and serve.

BREAKFASTS

PER SERVING
CALORIES: 89
TOTAL FAT: 3 G
SODIUM: 96 MG
CARBS: 16 G
SUGAR: 8 G
PROTEIN: 3 G

SWEET BROILED GRAPEFRUIT

KIDS' FAVORITE | QUICK + EASY

▸ Serves 4

▸ Prep time: 5 minutes ▸ Cook time: 5 minutes

Sometimes modest ingredients prepared simply can have impressive culinary impact. Tart, tangy grapefruit is incredibly juicy when broiled, and the light drizzle of honey creates a gorgeous caramelized top. Honey should be eaten in moderation on the Autoimmune Paleo Diet, and this easy breakfast is an ideal way to enjoy just a small amount of the natural sweetener.

2 red grapefruits
1 tablespoon local organic honey
½ teaspoon ground cinnamon

BREAKFASTS

1. Preheat the oven to broil.

2. Place an oven rack in the top position.

3. Cut the grapefruits in half and use a knife to loosen the segments from the membranes.

4. Place the grapefruit halves on a baking sheet, cut-side up, and drizzle the halves evenly with the honey.

5. Sprinkle the cinnamon over the honey.

6. Broil the grapefruits until they are lightly caramelized on top, about 5 minutes.

7. Serve one half per person.

PER SERVING
CALORIES 70
TOTAL FAT: 0 G
SODIUM: 0 MG
CARBS: 18 G
SUGAR: 15 G
PROTEIN: 1 G

BUTTERNUT SQUASH PORRIDGE

KIDS' FAVORITE | QUICK+EASY | GOOD FOR BATCHES

▶ Serves 4

▶ Prep time: 10 minutes ▶ Cook time: 10 minutes

If your idea of breakfast is a warm, lightly spiced bowl of oatmeal, you will certainly enjoy this filling substitute. The recipe will work with both boiled and baked squash as well as roasted vegetables. If you are making another recipe with squash, get an extra-large squash and purée the excess to use for this dish.

3 cups cooked butternut squash

1 apple, peeled, cored, and chopped

1 cup unsweetened organic coconut milk (for homemade, see page 258)

1 teaspoon ground cinnamon

½ teaspoon ground ginger

Pinch ground cloves

Pinch sea salt

1. Place the squash, apple, coconut milk, cinnamon, ginger, cloves, and salt in a food processor and pulse until smooth.

2. Transfer the squash mixture to a medium saucepan and place the pan over medium heat.

3. Heat the squash porridge, stirring often, until it is completely warmed through, about 10 minutes.

4. Serve immediately.

BREAKFASTS

PER SERVING
CALORIES: 85
TOTAL FAT: 1 G
SODIUM: 67 MG
CARBS: 19 G
SUGAR: 7 G
PROTEIN: 1 G

CELERIAC AND TURNIP PANCAKES

GOOD FOR BATCHES

- Serves 4
- Prep time: 20 minutes ▸ Cook time: 30 minutes

Celeriac and turnip, lightly accented with thyme and sweet carrot, are a perfect earthy combination with the applesauce. Celeriac might look like a strange hairy root, but it is packed with vitamins and nutrients that support a healthy immune system. Pastured lard is rendered from pasture-raised pigs and has not been hydrogenated. That gives it a shorter shelf life but an excellent health profile.

1 celeriac root, peeled and shredded (about 5 cups)

3 turnips, peeled and shredded (about 4 cups)

1 carrot, peeled and shredded (about 1 cup)

½ sweet onion, diced

2 tablespoons arrowroot powder

1 teaspoon chopped fresh thyme or ½ teaspoon dried thyme

½ teaspoon sea salt

¼ cup pastured lard

½ cup Spiced Applesauce (page 249)

PER SERVING

CALORIES: 243

TOTAL FAT: 13 G

SODIUM: 501 MG

CARBS: 30 G

SUGAR: 9 G

PROTEIN 4 G

1. Place the shredded celeriac, turnips, and carrot in a sieve and squeeze out as much liquid as possible. Discard the liquid.

2. Transfer the vegetables to a large bowl and add the onion, arrowroot, thyme, and salt, and stir until well combined.

3. Place a large skillet over medium heat and add the lard.

4. When the lard is melted and hot, add the shredded vegetable mixture, ¾ cup at a time, flattening each pancake with a spatula. Cook 4 pancakes at a time.

5. Cook the pancakes, flipping them carefully once, until they are golden and crispy, about 10 minutes.

6. Transfer the cooked pancakes to a paper towel–lined plate.

7. Repeat until all the shredded vegetable mixture is cooked and you have made about 12 pancakes.

8. Serve 3 pancakes per person, topping each serving with applesauce.

BREAKFAST COOKIES

▶ Makes 18 cookies

▶ Prep time: 10 minutes, plus 30 minutes to thicken ▶ Cook time: 20 minutes

Life can be hectic, and a convenient grab-and-go breakfast can save time and supply enough energy to tackle your morning. Dates provide some of the sweetness in these hearty cookies and are an easily digested source of healthy fiber. Dates do contain high levels of fructose, so these cookies are a wonderful way to get all the nutrients of the fruit in an acceptable portion size. Coconut flour sucks up moisture like a sponge, so you need a lot of wet ingredients. If you want to adapt a recipe you already have, for every cup of regular flour, you should substitute about ⅓ cup of coconut flour.

BREAKFASTS

PER SERVING
CALORIES: 84
TOTAL FAT: 6 G
SODIUM: 124 MG
CARBS: 8 G
SUGAR: 3 G
PROTEIN: 1 G

1½ cups mashed bananas (about 2)

¾ cup Spiced Applesauce (page 249)

3 tablespoons coconut oil

5 pitted dates

2 teaspoons freshly squeezed lime juice

¾ cup shredded unsweetened coconut

½ cup coconut flour

2 teaspoons ground cinnamon

1½ teaspoons baking soda

½ teaspoon ground ginger

Pinch ground cloves

Pinch sea salt

¼ cup dried cranberries

1. Preheat the oven to 350°F.

2. Line a baking sheet with parchment paper.

3. Place the bananas, applesauce, coconut oil, dates, and lime juice in a food processor or a blender and pulse until the mixture is very smooth, about 1 minute.

4. Add the shredded coconut, coconut flour, cinnamon, baking soda, ginger, cloves, and salt, and pulse until combined, about 1 minute.

5. Transfer the batter to a bowl and stir in the cranberries.

6. Let the batter sit for at least 30 minutes to thicken.

7. Drop the batter in heaps about the size of golf balls onto the baking sheet and flatten them out. Place the cookies relatively close together because they do not spread.

8. Bake the cookies until they are lightly golden and firm, about 20 minutes.

9. Cool the cookies completely on wire racks and store them in a sealed container at room temperature for up to 1 week.

BREAKFASTS

SWEET POTATO BREAKFAST CASSEROLE

MAKE AHEAD | GOOD FOR BATCHES

▸ Serves 4

▸ Prep time: 15 minutes ▸ Cook time: 1 hour, 40 minutes

Casseroles are a convenient, tasty option when you want an easy meal to prepare. You can make this casserole ahead of time and put it in the oven in the morning with little fuss. Simply leave out the coconut milk when you wrap the casserole up the night before, and pour the milk over it just before baking the dish.

1 tablespoon extra-virgin olive oil

1 sweet onion, thinly sliced

4 sweet potatoes (about 1¼ pounds), peeled and thinly sliced

1 pear, peeled, cored, and chopped

1 teaspoon sea salt

1 cup unsweetened organic coconut milk (for homemade, see page 258)

BREAKFASTS

PER SERVING
CALORIES: 265
TOTAL FAT: 5 G
SODIUM: 483 MG
CARBS: 55 G
SUGAR: 8 G
PROTEIN: 3 G

1. Preheat the oven to 350°F.

2. Place a large skillet over medium-high heat and add the olive oil.

3. Add the sliced onion and sauté until they are lightly caramelized, about 10 minutes.

4. While the onions are cooking, toss the sweet potatoes, pear, and salt in a large bowl.

5. Transfer one-third of the sweet potato mixture to a 9-by-13-inch baking dish and spread the mixture out evenly.

6. Top the sweet potato layer with half the cooked onions.

7. Repeat the layers, ending with the final one-third of the sweet potato mixture.

8. Pour the coconut milk evenly into the casserole.

9. Cover the casserole with foil and bake it for 1 hour.

10. Remove the foil and bake the casserole an additional 30 minutes, or until the potatoes are very tender.

11. Let the casserole sit for 10 minutes before serving.

STUFFED SQUASH

MAKE AHEAD | GOOD FOR BATCHES

▶ Serves 4

▶ Prep time: 15 minutes ▶ Cook time: 1 hour

Acorn squash is often an overlooked ingredient because it can be very difficult to cut open. This incredibly hard vegetable has firm, sweet flesh and is the perfect size for serving two people. If you want to cut your squash easily, try piercing the skin a few times with a fork and microwaving the squash for 2 minutes on high. Also, do not try to cut across the diameter of the squash; start at the stem end and cut right through to the other end.

2 acorn squash, halved and seeded

2 parsnips, peeled and finely chopped

1 pear, peeled, cored, and chopped

¼ cup dried cranberries

2 tablespoons raisins

2 teaspoons coconut oil or avocado oil

½ teaspoon ground cinnamon

Pinch ground cloves

Pinch ground ginger

Pinch sea salt

BREAKFASTS

PER SERVING
CALORIES: 177
TOTAL FAT: 1 G
SODIUM: 73 MG
CARBS: 45 G
SUGAR: 9 G
PROTEIN: 3 G

1. Preheat the oven to 375°F.

2. Place the squash halves cut-side down in a baking dish big enough to fit all of them.

3. Pour boiling water into the dish until it is ¼ inch deep. Bake the squash until tender, about 30 minutes.

4. While the squash is baking, stir the parsnips, pear, cranberries, raisins, coconut oil, cinnamon, cloves, ginger, and salt in a small bowl until well combined.

5. Remove the squash from the oven and pour any remaining water out of the baking dish. ▶

Stuffed Squash *continued*

6. Flip the squash over and divide the pear mixture evenly among the halves.

7. Return the filled squash to the oven and bake for an additional 25 to 30 minutes, until the squash is very tender.

8. Serve one half per person.

BREAKFASTS

BREAKFAST CHICKEN BURGERS

FODMAP-FREE | MAKE AHEAD | GOOD FOR BATCHES

▶ Serves 4

▶ Prep time: 10 minutes ▶ Cook time: 25 minutes

These burgers have no buns; instead, they use herbed chicken patties to hold together the crispy bacon, creamy avocado, and fresh lettuce fillings. You can use any Autoimmune Paleo Diet–approved ingredients to fill these meat sandwiches, such as olives, peaches, fresh herbs, and even coleslaw.

1 pound lean ground chicken

1 teaspoon chopped fresh basil or ½ teaspoon dried basil

1 teaspoon chopped fresh thyme or ½ teaspoon dried thyme

¼ teaspoon sea salt

8 slices organic bacon

1 avocado, peeled, pitted, and cut into 8 slices

4 lettuce leaves

1. Preheat the oven to 350°F.

2. Line a baking sheet with parchment paper.

3. Stir the chicken, basil, thyme, and salt in a medium mixing bowl until well combined.

4. Divide the chicken mixture into 8 equal pieces and form the pieces into ½-inch-thick patties.

5. Transfer the patties to the baking sheet and bake, turning once, until the patties are cooked through, about 20 minutes.

6. While the chicken patties are baking, cook the bacon in a small skillet over medium-high heat until crispy, about 5 minutes. Drain the bacon on a paper towel–lined plate.

7. Remove the cooked patties from the oven and use a paper towel to pat the excess fat from them.

8. Place the patties on a clean work surface and top 4 of the patties with 2 bacon slices, 2 avocado slices, and a leaf of lettuce each.

9. Top the stacks with a chicken patty each to form 4 burgers.

BREAKFASTS

PER SERVING

CALORIES: 339

TOTAL FAT: 22 G

SODIUM: 612 MG

CARBS: 5 G

SUGAR: 0 G

PROTEIN: 30 G

TURKEY BREAKFAST STIR-FRY

QUICK + EASY | GOOD FOR BATCHES

▸ Serves 4

▸ Prep time: 15 minutes ▸ Cook time: 15 minutes

This stir-fry is a wonderful transition recipe from traditional breakfasts foods because it is packed with tender-crisp vegetables and small chunks of savory and satisfying turkey. When following the Autoimmune Paleo Diet, it is important to find the highest-quality meats possible, and turkey is no exception. You won't find grass-fed birds, because turkeys are omnivores and their food is supplemented with feed, seeds, and sometimes even table scraps. The best choice for turkeys is organic pasture-raised, which means they are allowed to roam freely and are not given antibiotics.

PER SERVING
CALORIES: 190
TOTAL FAT: 10 G
SODIUM: 613 MG
CARBS: 15 G
SUGAR: 6 G
PROTEIN: 13 G

2 tablespoons coconut oil

2 cups broccoli florets

1 parsnip, peeled and chopped

1 carrot, peeled and sliced

1 celery stalk, sliced

1 cup sliced mushrooms

8 ounces cooked turkey breast, chopped

1 teaspoon minced fresh garlic

1 teaspoon grated fresh ginger

1 cup shredded spinach

¼ cup shredded unsweetened coconut

1. Place a large skillet over medium-high heat and add the coconut oil.

2. When the oil is hot, add the broccoli, parsnip, and carrot, and stir-fry the vegetables until they are tender-crisp, about 4 minutes.

3. Add the celery and mushrooms and stir-fry the vegetables until they are tender, another 4 minutes.

4. Add the turkey, garlic, and ginger, and stir until fragrant and the turkey is warmed through, about 4 minutes.

5. Add the spinach and stir until wilted, about 2 minutes.

6. Divide the stir-fry among 4 plates and serve topped with the coconut.

SIMPLE PORK SAUSAGE

MAKE AHEAD | KIDS' FAVORITE | QUICK+EASY | GOOD FOR BATCHES

▸ Serves 4

▸ Prep time: 10 minutes ▸ Cook time: 16 minutes

Sausage is a familiar breakfast food, even when it is not cozied up to a couple of sunny-side up eggs. These homemade patties are fragrant with garlic and parsley, but any Autoimmune Paleo Diet herb or spice will work well. You can double this recipe and freeze the extra cooked patties for a quick protein-packed meal. Just take the patties out of the freezer the night before and thaw them in the refrigerator for the next day.

1 pound ground pork

1½ teaspoons minced fresh garlic

1 teaspoon dried minced onion

1 tablespoon chopped fresh parsley or 1 teaspoon dried parsley

½ teaspoon sea salt

3 teaspoons extra-virgin olive oil

1. Mix the pork, garlic, onion, parsley, and salt in a large bowl until well combined.

2. Divide the pork into 8 pieces and form the pieces into ½-inch-thick patties.

3. Place a large skillet over medium-high heat and add 1½ teaspoons of olive oil.

4. Fry 4 patties until they are cooked through and golden, about 4 minutes per side, then transfer them to a paper towel–lined plate.

5. Add the remaining 1½ teaspoons of olive oil and fry the other 4 patties the same way.

6. Serve 2 patties per person.

BREAKFASTS

PER SERVING

CALORIES: 195

TOTAL FAT: 7 G

SODIUM: 299 MG

CARBS: 1 G

SUGAR: 0 G

PROTEIN: 30 G

SWEET POTATO BACON HASH BROWNS

▸ Serves 4

▸ Prep time: 15 minutes ▸ Cook time: 20 minutes

Hash browns are often a side to breakfast, but these golden bacon-studded patties deserve center stage. The soft, almost creamy center is a pleasing contrast to the crisp exterior. Sweet potatoes are an ideal substitute for most dishes that typically use white potatoes. Arrowroot powder is the dried ground-up roots of the arrowroot plant. It is used as a thickener and is gluten-free as well as flavorless. It contains omega-3 fatty acids and is a good source of calcium and potassium.

3 sweet potatoes (about 1 pound), peeled and cut into 1-inch chunks

5 slices organic bacon, chopped

2 scallions, chopped

1 tablespoon arrowroot powder

1 teaspoon chopped fresh thyme or ½ teaspoon dried thyme

2 teaspoons extra-virgin olive oil

BREAKFASTS

PER SERVING
CALORIES: 381
TOTAL FAT: 13 G
SODIUM: 321 MG
CARBS: 55 G
SUGAR: 1 G
PROTEIN: 12 G

1. Place the sweet potatoes in a large saucepan, cover the potatoes with water, and place the saucepan over medium-high heat.

2. Bring the sweet potatoes to a boil, then reduce the heat to low and simmer the potatoes until they are tender, about 10 minutes.

3. While the potatoes are simmering, cook the chopped bacon in a large skillet over medium-high heat until crispy, about 5 minutes. Drain the bacon on a paper towel–lined plate. Wipe the skillet out and set aside.

4. Drain the sweet potatoes and mash them, leaving them slightly chunky.

5. Add the cooked bacon, scallions, arrowroot, and thyme to the potatoes, and stir to combine. Set the mixture aside for 10 minutes to firm up.

6. Form the sweet potato mixture into 4 equal patties.

7. Place the reserved large skillet over medium-high heat and add the olive oil.

8. Fry the sweet potato patties until they are golden brown and crispy on the outside, turning once, about 3 minutes per side.

9. Serve 1 patty per person.

BREAKFAST "PIZZA"

MAKE AHEAD | KIDS' FAVORITE | QUICK+EASY | GOOD FOR BATCHES

▸ Serves 4

▸ Prep time: 15 minutes ▸ Cook time: 15 minutes

A thin cooked meat layer makes a marvelous base for tasty toppings on this "pizza," minus the bread crust. The toppings in this recipe are just a suggestion, so try your favorite vegetables and fermented foods for a dish that's just the way you like it. You can even spread the meat crust with Tomato-Free "Marinara" Sauce (page 107) for a simple, tasty breakfast. The meat "crust" mixture can be doubled and even tripled so that you can take advantage of a ground beef sale at your local grocery store. Simply make the recipe and divide the meat mixture into pizza portions. Freeze the extra portions in sealed plastic bags for up to three months, labeled with the date and contents.

2 pounds lean ground beef

3 teaspoons chopped fresh thyme or 1½ teaspoons dried thyme

2 teaspoons minced fresh garlic

1 tablespoon chopped fresh oregano or 1 teaspoon dried oregano

1 teaspoon dried minced onion

1 teaspoon sea salt

2½ cups assorted chopped vegetables and other favorite toppings
(good choices: artichokes, asparagus, broccoli, leeks, mushrooms, cooked sweet potato, and olives)

1. Preheat the oven to 450°F.

2. Line a 9-by-13-inch rimmed baking sheet with parchment paper and set aside.

3. Mix the ground beef, thyme, garlic, oregano, onion, and salt in a large bowl until well combined.

4. Transfer the meat mixture to the baking sheet and spread it out so it covers as much of the pan as possible, about ½ inch thick.

5. Bake the meat until it is cooked through, about 10 minutes, then remove it from the oven. ▸

BREAKFASTS

PER SERVING

CALORIES: 458

TOTAL FAT: 14 G

SODIUM: 658 MG

CARBS: 7 G

SUGAR: 1 G

PROTEIN: 71 G

Breakfast "Pizza" *continued*

6. Turn the oven to broil.

7. Carefully pour out the excess grease from the baking sheet and use a paper towel to blot the top of the meat.

8. Top the meat crust evenly with the toppings you have chosen so that the toppings form a generous layer.

9. Broil the pizza until the toppings are tender and lightly browned, about 5 minutes.

10. Remove the pizza from the oven, cut it into 4 portions, and serve.

BREAKFASTS

PUMPKIN AND GROUND BEEF HASH

MAKE AHEAD | GOOD FOR BATCHES

- ► Serves 4
- ► Prep time: 10 minutes ► Cook time: 25 minutes

Pumpkin is considered a fall vegetable, but it can be purchased year-round. The pumpkin adds a slightly sweet taste and glorious sunny color to this dish that is enhanced by the addition of turmeric. If you can only get a large pumpkin, cut the unused portion into chunks and freeze them on a baking tray. When the chunks are frozen, transfer them to a sealable plastic bag and freeze them for up to 3 months.

1½ pounds lean ground beef

1 sweet onion, chopped

2 teaspoons minced fresh garlic

1 pumpkin (about 2 pounds), peeled, cooked, and diced

1 teaspoon ground ginger

½ teaspoon turmeric

¼ teaspoon sea salt

Pinch ground cloves

1 cup spinach

BREAKFASTS

PER SERVING
CALORIES: 384
TOTAL FAT: 11 G
SODIUM: 237 MG
CARBS: 16 G
SUGAR: 4 G
PROTEIN: 54 G

1. Place a large skillet over medium-high heat and add the ground beef.

2. Sauté the meat until it is no longer pink, about 10 minutes.

3. Add the onion and garlic and sauté for 2 minutes.

4. Add the pumpkin, ginger, turmeric, salt, and cloves, and reduce the heat to medium.

5. Cook, stirring, until the pumpkin breaks down and is heated through, about 10 minutes.

6. Add the spinach and stir until it is wilted, about 3 minutes.

7. Divide the beef mixture into 4 bowls and serve.

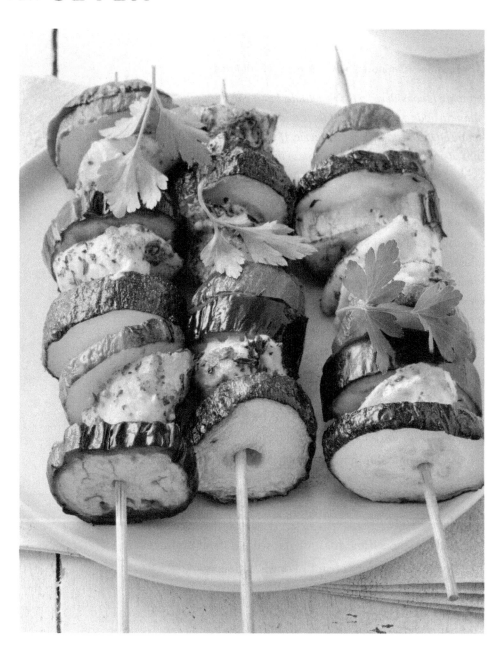

SNACKS

HONEYDEW ICE POPS

MAKE AHEAD | KIDS' FAVORITE | QUICK+EASY | GOOD FOR BATCHES

- ▸ Makes 8 ice pops (1 ice pop per serving)
- ▸ Prep time: 10 minutes, plus 4 hours to chill

Honeydew melons are a member of the gourd family, just like pumpkin and squash, and are packed with vitamin C and low in calories. For a perfect sweet honeydew, look for a melon that is heavy for its size with a waxy skin that does not stay indented when you press on it. Taste your melon before adding the honey in this recipe, because you might find it sweet enough. Honey is allowed in moderation on the Autoimmune Paleo Diet because it is unrefined. Honey also has beneficial anti-inflammatory and antioxidant properties as well as minerals such as iron, potassium, and calcium. If you are FODMAP intolerant, the high fructose in honey could be an issue, so exclude it from this recipe.

½ honeydew melon (about 1 pound), peeled, seeded, and diced

½ cup water

Juice of 1 lime

1 teaspoon local organic honey

Pinch sea salt

1. Place the honeydew and water in a blender and pulse until the melon is smooth, about 1 minute.

2. Add the lime juice, honey, and salt, and pulse to combine.

3. Pour the melon mixture into ice pop molds and freeze for about 4 hours, until firm.

SNACKS

PER SERVING

CALORIES: 26

TOTAL FAT: 0 G

SODIUM: 42 MG

CARBS: 6 G

SUGAR: 6 G

PROTEIN: 1 G

LEMON-RASPBERRY MUFFINS

FODMAP-FREE | KIDS' FAVORITE | GOOD FOR BATCHES

▸ Makes 18 muffins (1 muffin per serving)
▸ Prep time: 20 minutes, plus 1 hour to chill ▸ Cook time: 25 minutes

These cheerful berry beauties have a firm cheesecake texture and distinctive tart-sweet flavor. Raspberries are one of the most perishable fruits, so they should be stored in the refrigerator at all times and eaten within a couple days of purchase. To get the full impact of the antioxidants in raspberries, eat them when they are completely ripe because that is when the antioxidant support is highest. You can also use blueberries or cut-up strawberries in these muffins, for a different taste.

4½ cups shredded unsweetened coconut
¾ cup maple syrup
Juice and zest of 1 lemon
1 teaspoon baking soda
Pinch sea salt
¾ cup raspberries

1. Preheat the oven to 350°F.

2. Line 18 muffin cups with paper liners and set aside.

3. Place the coconut in a food processor or a blender and process until it is semi-liquid, scraping down the sides, about 10 minutes.

4. Add the maple syrup and lemon juice and zest, and process the batter for 2 minutes.

5. Add the baking soda and salt and process until combined, about 30 seconds.

6. Pour the batter into the muffin cups and evenly divide the raspberries among the muffins, pressing them into the batter.

7. Bake the muffins until they are lightly golden, 20 to 25 minutes.

8. Remove the muffins from the oven and let them stand for 10 minutes.

9. Chill the muffins in the refrigerator for at least 1 hour before serving.

10. Store leftover muffins in a sealed container in the refrigerator for up to 5 days.

SNACKS

PER SERVING
CALORIES: 237
TOTAL FAT: 18 G
SODIUM: 94 MG
CARBS: 19 G
SUGAR: 10 G
PROTEIN: 2 G

SPICED PEAR CHIPS

- ▸ Makes 8 servings
- ▸ Prep time: 10 minutes ▸ Cook time: 2 hours

These chips, with their hint of salt to intensify the sweetness of the pear, are addictive. The best time to eat them is right after they are cool, because they can soften a little as they sit and become more like a fruit leather. The best way to get very thin, uniform slices is to use a mandoline. This handy kitchen tool has an assortment of blades that produce slices, crosshatch patterns, ribbons, sticks, and batons.

3 pears, cored and very thinly sliced
½ teaspoon ground cinnamon
Pinch sea salt

SNACKS

PER SERVING
CALORIES: 46
TOTAL FAT: 0 G
SODIUM: 32 MG
CARBS: 12 G
SUGAR: 7 G
PROTEIN: 0 G

1. Preheat the oven to 225°F.

2. Line 2 baking sheets with parchment paper.

3. Spread the pear slices on the baking sheets with no overlap.

4. Sprinkle the slices with the cinnamon and sea salt.

5. Place the baking sheets in the oven and bake until the chips are crisp and dry, turning once, about 2 hours.

6. Remove the chips from the oven and let them cool before serving.

7. Store the chips in a sealed container at room temperature for up to 3 days.

EASY APPLE BUTTER

▸ Makes 4 cups (2 tablespoons per serving)
▸ Prep time: 15 minutes ▸ Cook time: 5 to 6 hours

As apples slowly cook down, they take on a velvety, rich texture. This slow-cooker method is the simplest way to make apple butter, but you can also cook this spread in a large pot on the stove over low heat, cooking for about 3 hours, and get very similar results. If you are using the stove-top method, make sure you stir the apples every 30 minutes or so.

5 pounds apples, peeled, cored, and chopped
½ cup water
¼ cup freshly squeezed lemon juice
1 tablespoon ground cinnamon
½ teaspoon ground ginger
¼ teaspoon ground cloves

1. Place the apples, water, and lemon juice in a slow cooker set to low and cook until the apples are very tender, stirring occasionally, about 5 hours.

2. Transfer the apples to a blender and add the cinnamon, ginger, and cloves.

3. Blend until the mixture is smooth and buttery, about 4 minutes.

4. Transfer the apple mixture back to the slow cooker and cook on high without the lid until the mixture is thick, about 45 minutes.

5. Cool the apple butter completely and store it in a sealed container in the refrigerator for up to 2 weeks.

6. Serve the butter with Autoimmune Paleo Diet–approved cookies or cut-up vegetables.

SNACKS

PER SERVING
CALORIES: 19
TOTAL FAT: 0 G
SODIUM: 1 MG
CARBS: 5 G
SUGAR: 4 G
PROTEIN: 0 G

SPICED PEACH SPREAD

MAKE AHEAD | KIDS' FAVORITE | GOOD FOR BATCHES

▸ Makes 4 cups (2 tablespoons per serving)
▸ Prep time: 20 minutes ▸ Cook time: 1 hour

Ripe peaches are the embodiment of summer. The lush, sweet scent and sunrise hue of their skin seems almost decadent. This peach spread seems to distill all that goodness down into an intense, smooth indulgence. Do not worry if there does not seem to be enough liquid when you first start cooking your peach mixture; the fruit will purge juice as it cooks.

4 pounds peaches, pitted and coarsely chopped
¼ cup freshly squeezed lemon juice
1 teaspoon ground cinnamon
Pinch ground cloves

PER SERVING
CALORIES: 28
TOTAL FAT 1 G
SODIUM: 0 MG
CARBS: 7 G
SUGAR: 6 G
PROTEIN: 1 G

1. Purée the chopped peaches in a food processor or a blender and transfer them to a large saucepan.

2. Add the lemon juice, cinnamon, and cloves to the peaches and place the saucepan over medium heat.

3. Cook the peach mixture, stirring frequently, until it starts to simmer, then reduce the heat to low.

4. Simmer the peach mixture until it thickens and reduces by a third, about 1 hour.

5. Remove the saucepan from the heat and pour the peach spread into a container.

6. Cool the spread to room temperature and store it, covered, in the refrigerator for up to 1 week.

7. Serve the spread with fruit or Autoimmune Paleo Diet–approved cookies.

CARAMEL-COCONUT DIP

FODMAP-FREE | MAKE AHEAD | KIDS' FAVORITE | QUICK+EASY | GOOD FOR BATCHES

▸ Makes 2 cups (2 tablespoons per serving)

▸ Prep time: 10 minutes

This dip is perfect when you need something spectacular in a pinch. It whips together in no time at all and tastes like you spent hours slaving over a hot stove. Although any grade of maple syrup will work well, the best choice for this luscious dip is grade B or a darker, richer syrup to get a true caramel flavor.

1 tablespoon coconut oil, melted

3 cups shredded unsweetened coconut

¼ cup maple syrup

⅛ teaspoon sea salt

1. Place the coconut oil, coconut, maple syrup, and salt in a blender and blend the ingredients until smooth and buttery, about 4 minutes.

2. Transfer the dip to a sealed container and store it at room temperature for up to 5 days.

3. Serve the dip with fruit.

SNACKS

PER SERVING

CALORIES 73

TOTAL FAT: 6 G

SODIUM: 19 MG

CARBS: 6 G

SUGAR: 4 G

PROTEIN: 1 G

HERBED MUSHROOM PÂTÉ

▸ Serves 8

▸ Prep time: 10 minutes ▸ Cook time: 15 minutes

Pâté is usually puréed liver, but this silky, thick mushroom-based pâté proves that a fungi can also be a spectacular spread. Any mushroom will work well, but shitakes add an incredibly rich, earthy flavor and meaty texture to the dish. If you want to use portobello mushrooms, make sure you scoop the dark gills out so that your pâté is a more appetizing color. Shiitake mushrooms should be available in most grocery stores, but if you can't find them, try a local Asian market. You can store shiitake mushrooms up to one week in the refrigerator in a sealed paper bag. Avoid mushrooms that have any damp or soft spots on them; they should be dry and firm.

SNACKS

PER SERVING
CALORIES: 110
TOTAL FAT: 6 G
SODIUM: 77 MG
CARBS: 12 G
SUGAR: 4 G
PROTEIN: 2 G

¼ cup extra-virgin olive oil

1 cup stemmed shiitake mushrooms

1 cup sliced brown button mushrooms

2 cups shredded sweet potato

1 sweet onion, finely chopped

1 tablespoon chopped fresh thyme or 1 teaspoon dried thyme

½ teaspoon chopped fresh tarragon or ¼ teaspoon dried tarragon

¼ teaspoon sea salt

1. Place a large skillet over medium-high heat and add the olive oil.

2. Sauté the shiitake mushrooms, brown button mushrooms, sweet potato, and onion until the fungi and vegetables are tender and cooked, about 10 minutes.

3. Add the thyme, tarragon, and salt, and sauté for 5 minutes.

4. Transfer the mushroom mixture to a food processor or a blender and pulse until the mixture is smooth, scraping down the sides, about 3 minutes.

5. Transfer the mixture to a container and allow it to cool to room temperature, about 45 minutes.

6. Seal the container and store in the refrigerator for up to 1 week.

ENDIVE BOATS

MAKE AHEAD | QUICK+EASY | GOOD FOR BATCHES

- ▶ Makes 12 boats (1 boat per serving)
- ▶ Prep time: 15 minutes

These easy-to-prepare stuffed creations are the perfect choice if you need a fancy appetizer for a special event. If you cannot find BPA-free cans of tuna, you can also chop up fresh cooked tuna or use cooked chicken. BPA, or bisphenol A, is an industrial chemical that can leach into food from plastics and the lining of cans. BPA exposure is the subject of many studies concerning autoimmune diseases such as type 1 diabetes.

1 (5-ounce) BPA-free can water-packed tuna, drained
1 carrot, peeled and shredded
1 celery stalk, diced
1 Naturally Fermented Pickle (page 262), finely chopped
2 tablespoons freshly squeezed lemon juice
½ teaspoon minced fresh garlic
Pinch sea salt
2 endive heads, separated into leaves

PER SERVING
CALORIES: 33
TOTAL FAT: 1 G
SODIUM: 97 MG
CARBS: 4 G
SUGAR: 1 G
PROTEIN: 4 G

1. Mix the tuna, carrot, celery, pickle, lemon juice, garlic, and salt in a small bowl until well combined.

2. Pick out 12 large endive leaves and spoon the tuna salad into the leaves. Use the extra endive leaves for another recipe.

3. Store the endive boats covered in plastic wrap in the refrigerator for up to 2 days.

CHICKEN SALAD LETTUCE CUPS

KIDS' FAVORITE | QUICK+EASY | GOOD FOR BATCHES

▸ Serves 4
▸ Prep time: 15 minutes

Crispy lettuce and cabbage leaves make an effective wrap for tasty fillings. The jicama and celery in the chicken salad give it a satisfying, crisp crunch, and the grapes provide an interesting, sweet counterpoint. Jicama can help support a healthy immune system and has excellent disease-fighting antioxidant and anti-inflammatory properties.

1 pound cooked chicken breast, chopped
1 celery stalk, finely diced
½ cup peeled and shredded carrot
½ cup halved red grapes
½ cup finely chopped jicama
¼ cup chopped sweet onion
½ teaspoon chopped fresh tarragon or ¼ teaspoon dried tarragon
Pinch sea salt
8 lettuce leaves

1. Mix the chicken, celery, carrot, grapes, jicama, onion, tarragon, and salt in a medium bowl until well combined.

2. Divide the chicken salad evenly between the lettuce leaves and serve.

SNACKS

PER SERVING
CALORIES: 216
TOTAL FAT: 4 G
SODIUM: 204 MG
CARBS: 7 G
SUGAR: 4 G
PROTEIN: 37 G

CHICKEN AND ZUCCHINI KEBABS

FODMAP-FREE | QUICK+EASY

▸ Serves 4

▸ Prep time: 15 minutes ▸ Cook time: 10 minutes

Kebabs are fun and exotic-looking, despite the absolute simplicity of their preparation. What could be easier than spearing meats and vegetables on a stick? Zucchini is high in vitamins A and C, which are crucial for immune system support, as well as potassium, which is heart-friendly. Try using both green and yellow squash for a lovely-looking kebab.

1 green or yellow zucchini, cut into 10 chunks

1 long purple eggplant, cut into 10 slices

2 (8-ounce) boneless, skinless chicken breasts, cut into 8 chunks each

1 teaspoon extra-virgin olive oil

1 teaspoon dried oregano

Dash sea salt

Juice of 1 lemon

1. Soak 4 wooden skewers in water for 30 minutes.

2. Skewer 5 zucchini chunks and eggplant and 4 chicken chunks onto each wooden skewer.

3. Brush the kebabs with olive oil and sprinkle them with oregano and salt.

4. Preheat the barbecue to medium-high heat and place the lemon juice in a small bowl beside the barbecue with a brush.

5. Grill the kebabs for about 10 minutes, turning to cook all the sides, or until cooked through. Brush the lemon juice over the kebabs before the last 2 minutes of cooking.

6. If you do not have a barbecue, preheat the oven to broil and place a wire rack on a baking sheet. Lay the kebabs on the wire rack and broil them for about 6 minutes per side, until the chicken is cooked through. Brush the kebabs with lemon juice when you turn them.

7. Serve warm.

SNACKS

PER SERVING
CALORIES: 260
TOTAL FAT: 10 G
SODIUM: 98 MG
CARBS: 8 G
SUGAR: 4 G
PROTEIN: 34 G

COCONUT CHICKEN FINGERS

KIDS' FAVORITE | QUICK+EASY | GOOD FOR BATCHES

▸ Serves 4

▸ Prep time: 15 minutes ▸ Cook time: 12 minutes

Kids in particular love chicken fingers, nuggets, and dinosaurs on their plate, but it is often difficult to determine what they are eating, and if it is really chicken. This dish is 100 percent lean chicken breast coated in a crispy coconut breading, and it is delicious. Coconut comes from palm trees, which are called "the tree of life" by Pacific cultures due to their medicinal and nutritional properties. Coconut is fabulous for the immune system because it can kill parasites, fungi, viruses, and bacteria.

SNACKS

PER SERVING
CALORIES: 453
TOTAL FAT: 29 G
SODIUM: 123 MG
CARBS: 14 G
SUGAR: 2 G
PROTEIN: 34 G

4 tablespoons arrowroot powder

⅛ teaspoon sea salt

½ cup unsweetened organic coconut milk (for homemade, see page 258)

1 cup shredded unsweetened coconut

2 (8-ounce) boneless, skinless chicken breasts, cut into 6 strips lengthwise

2 tablespoons extra-virgin olive oil

1. Preheat the oven to 400°F.

2. Line a baking sheet with parchment paper and set aside.

3. Mix the arrowroot and salt in a small bowl.

4. Pour the coconut milk into a small bowl.

5. Place the shredded coconut on a plate.

6. Pat the chicken strips dry with a paper towel.

7. Dredge a chicken strip in the arrowroot mixture, dip it into the coconut milk, and then dredge it in the shredded coconut. Place the coated strip on the baking sheet.

8. Repeat this breading process with all the chicken.

9. Lightly brush the strips with olive oil.

10. Bake the chicken until it is cooked through and the coconut coating is golden, turning once, about 12 minutes total.

11. Serve warm.

TURKEY SLIDERS

KIDS' FAVORITE | QUICK+EASY | GOOD FOR BATCHES

▸ Makes 12 sliders (3 sliders per serving)
▸ Prep time: 15 minutes ▸ Cook time: 10 minutes

When buying the turkey for these juicy little burgers, it is important to find organic, pasture-raised turkey. These birds are usually fed contaminant-free feed, and their meat has a higher nutrition profile. It might be a good idea to talk to local food–advocacy groups, who can point you toward organic farms in your area for all your meat and produce needs.

1 pound ground turkey
¼ cup chopped red onion
¼ cup chopped fresh parsley
1 teaspoon chopped fresh thyme or ½ teaspoon dried thyme
¼ teaspoon sea salt
1 tablespoon coconut oil or bacon fat

1. Mix the turkey, onion, parsley, thyme, and salt in a medium bowl until well combined.

2. Form the turkey mixture into 12 small burger patties.

3. Place a large skillet over medium-high heat and add the coconut oil.

4. Fry the turkey burgers until they are browned on both sides and cooked through, turning once, about 4 minutes per side.

5. Remove the sliders from the heat and pat off any excess oil with a paper towel.

6. Serve the sliders topped with Traditional Coleslaw (page 175).

SNACKS

PER SERVING
CALORIES: 354
TOTAL FAT: 23 G
SODIUM: 236 MG
CARBS: 10 G
SUGAR: 0 G
PROTEIN: 32 G

PORK AND VEGGIE MEATBALLS

MAKE AHEAD | KIDS' FAVORITE | GOOD FOR BATCHES

- ▸ Makes 24 meatballs (2 meatballs per serving)
- ▸ Prep time: 20 minutes ▸ Cook time: 30 minutes

Meatballs are found in almost every culture in the world; records describing this humble collection of minced meat and herbs date back to the year AD 25 in ancient Rome. This version has a hearty portion of added vegetables to provide healthy fiber and flavor. A couple of meatballs make a great snack, but these would also be superb combined with Tomato-Free "Marinara" Sauce (page 107) and long, fresh zucchini noodles for a family dinner. Basil is extremely perishable, so if you have any leftover, make a nice pesto or purée it and freeze it in ice cube trays for later use. Wrap the frozen basil cubes in plastic wrap. You can later simply unwrap and add the frozen cubes to soups, stews, and sauces.

SNACKS

PER SERVING
CALORIES: 84
TOTAL FAT: 4 G
SODIUM: 53 MG
CARBS: 1 G
SUGAR: 0 G
PROTEIN: 10 G

1 pound ground pork
1 pound ground turkey
1 cup shredded zucchini, with the liquid squeezed out
½ cup peeled and shredded carrot, with the liquid squeezed out
½ cup peeled and shredded parsnip, with the liquid squeezed out
2 tablespoons chopped fresh basil or 1 tablespoon dried basil
1 tablespoon minced fresh garlic
1 teaspoon grated fresh ginger
1 teaspoon chopped fresh cilantro
¼ teaspoon sea salt
3 tablespoons extra-virgin olive oil

1. Mix the pork, turkey, zucchini, carrot, parsnip, basil, garlic, ginger, cilantro, and salt in a large bowl and until well combined.

2. Form the mixture into about 24 golf ball–size meatballs.

3. Heat the olive oil in a large skillet over medium-high heat and add the meatballs in 2 batches.

4. Brown the meatballs on all sides until they are cooked through, about 15 minutes for each batch.

5. Serve warm or cold.

APPLE-BACON POPPERS

FODMAP-FREE | MAKE AHEAD | KIDS' FAVORITE | QUICK+EASY | GOOD FOR BATCHES

▸ Makes 16 poppers (2 poppers per serving)
▸ Prep time: 10 minutes ▸ Cook time: 5 minutes

Commercially packaged bacon can contain nitrates and sugar, so it is important to buy good-quality, sugar-free, pasture-raised pork bacon. You can also get pork belly from pastured pig from a reputable butcher and simply salt and spice it yourself before cooking it. This recipe would also be delicious with pear or melon instead of apple.

2 tart apples, peeled, cored, and cut into 8 pieces
1 tablespoon freshly squeezed lemon juice
4 slices organic bacon, cut into 2-inch pieces (about 16 pieces total)

1. Place the apple slices and lemon juice in a small bowl and toss so the apple is coated with lemon juice.

2. Place a large skillet over medium-high heat and fry the bacon pieces until they are just cooked through but not overly crisp, about 5 minutes.

3. Transfer the bacon to a paper towel–lined plate and blot the excess fat.

4. Place 1 apple slice between 2 pieces of bacon and secure it with a toothpick.

5. Repeat until all the apple slices and bacon are used.

6. Serve immediately.

SNACKS

PER SERVING
CALORIES: 22
TOTAL FAT: 1 G
SODIUM: 42 MG
CARBS: 3 G
SUGAR: 2 G
PROTEIN: 1 G

HONEY-THYME BEEF JERKY

MAKE AHEAD | GOOD FOR BATCHES

- ▶ Serves 8
- ▶ Prep time: 30 minutes, plus 2 to 6 hours to marinate
- ▶ Cook time: 8 to 10 hours

The beef jerky offered in most stores is usually packed with preservatives and nitrates and does not resemble meat at all anymore. This homemade version has a strong beef flavor and an interesting chewy texture. To get very thin strips of beef, try placing the raw meat in the freezer until it is semi-frozen before slicing it.

3 tablespoons apple cider vinegar

2 tablespoons local organic honey

2 tablespoons water

½ teaspoon sea salt

1 teaspoon garlic powder

1 teaspoon dried thyme

2 pounds beef, such as London broil

1. Mix the vinegar, honey, water, salt, garlic powder, and thyme in a large bowl until well combined. Set aside.

2. Slice the beef very thinly across the grain, about ⅛ inch thick.

3. Transfer the meat slices to the bowl of marinade. Toss to coat the meat slices and place the bowl in the refrigerator for 2 to 6 hours.

4. Remove the meat from the refrigerator and lay the strips on a paper towel–lined plate and pat them dry.

5. Line a large baking tray with foil and place it on the bottom rack of the oven. Move the top rack to the highest position.

6. Thread the beef pieces about 1 inch from one end of the strip onto wooden skewers so that each skewer has about 7 pieces dangling from it.

7. Set the skewers onto the top rack in the oven so that the beef strips dangle down between the rack bars.

PER SERVING

CALORIES: 229

TOTAL FAT: 7 G

SODIUM: 140 MG

CARBS: 5 G

SUGAR: 4 G

PROTEIN: 35 G

8. Repeat this process until all the beef strips are in the oven.

9. Turn on the oven to between 180°F and 200°F.

10. Prop the oven door open about 2 inches and cook the jerky until it is dry, about 8 to 10 hours.

11. Remove the jerky from the skewers and let it cool completely.

12. Store the jerky in a sealed container in the refrigerator for up to 1 month.

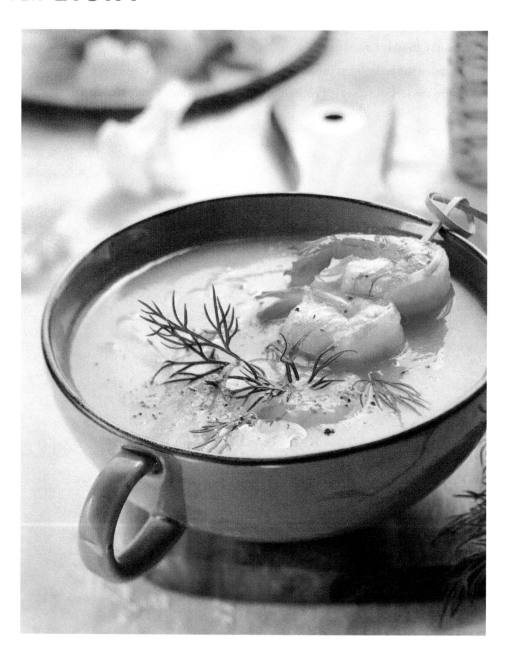

SOUPS AND STEWS

FENNEL-APPLE SOUP

▶ Serves 4

▶ Prep time: 15 minutes ▶ Cook time: 30 minutes

This soup is a delicate pale-green dish that is very spring-like in flavor and presentation. The subtle licorice taste of the fennel marries perfectly with the thyme and apple to create a special soup perfect for company. The sweetness of this soup depends entirely on what type of apples you use, so choose from tart Granny Smith to almost sugary Fuji apples to suit your palate. Make sure you save the feathery fennel fronds for an elegant garnish.

SOUPS AND STEWS

PER SERVING
CALORIES: 182
TOTAL FAT: 7 G
SODIUM: 230 MG
CARBS: 29 G
SUGAR: 7 G
PROTEIN: 3 G

2 tablespoons extra-virgin olive oil

½ sweet onion, chopped

1 teaspoon minced fresh garlic

3 fennel bulbs, stems and fronds removed, diced

2 celery stalks, chopped

1 apple (about ½ pound), peeled, cored, and diced

6 cups Chicken Bone Broth (page 266)

1 tablespoon chopped fresh thyme or 1 teaspoon dried thyme

¼ teaspoon sea salt

1. Place a large saucepan over medium heat and add the olive oil.

2. Sauté the onion and garlic until they are soft and lightly browned, about 5 minutes.

3. Add the fennel bulb, celery, and apple, and sauté until softened, about 8 minutes.

4. Add the chicken broth and thyme and bring the soup to a boil.

5. Reduce the heat to low and simmer until the vegetables and fruit are tender, about 15 minutes.

6. Transfer the mixture to a food processor or a blender and process until the soup is smooth, or use an immersion blender right in the pan.

7. Season with salt and serve.

SUNNY CARROT SOUP

MAKE AHEAD | KIDS' FAVORITE | GOOD FOR BATCHES

▶ Serves 4

▶ Prep time: 15 minutes ▶ Cook time: 25 minutes

Carrots are a spectacular source of beta-carotene, vitamins A and K, and fiber. These nutrients boost the immune system, protect against cardiovascular disease, and cut the risk of eye diseases such as glaucoma. This soup might become a staple lunch or light dinner to access all those nutrients. In the summer, carrot soup is also delicious cold.

2 tablespoons extra-virgin olive oil

½ sweet onion, chopped

1 tablespoon grated fresh ginger

1 teaspoon minced fresh garlic

1 teaspoon turmeric

6 cups Chicken Bone Broth (page 266)

1½ pounds carrots, peeled and chopped

1 sweet potato, peeled and chopped

1 cup unsweetened organic coconut milk (for homemade, see page 258)

2 tablespoons freshly squeezed lemon juice

¼ teaspoon sea salt

SOUPS AND STEWS

PER SERVING
CALORIES: 212
TOTAL FAT: 8 G
SODIUM: 140 MG
CARBS: 33 G
SUGAR: 11 G
PROTEIN: 3 G

1. Place a large saucepan over medium-high heat and add the olive oil.

2. Sauté the onion, ginger, garlic, and turmeric until the onion is soft, about 3 minutes.

3. Add the chicken broth, carrots, and sweet potato.

4. Bring the soup to a boil, then reduce the heat to low and simmer until the carrots are tender, about 20 minutes.

5. Transfer the soup to a food processor or blender, add the coconut milk, and process until the soup is smooth.

6. Add the lemon juice and salt and pulse to combine.

7. Serve warm.

FRENCH ONION SOUP

MAKE AHEAD | GOOD FOR BATCHES

▸ Serves 4

▸ Prep time: 10 minutes ▸ Cook time: 2 hours, 50 minutes

The process for making perfect French onion soup is much discussed among professional chefs. Flawlessly caramelized onions are required to produce the rich flavor of this traditional dish. Any onion will caramelize, but red onions tend to turn an unappetizing muddy green, so use them as a last resort. If you do not mind your caramelized onions a little soft, there is a quick way to get them golden. Add about ¼ teaspoon of baking soda per pound of onions right at the beginning of the cooking process, and you will have browned onions after about 10 minutes of sautéing.

SOUPS AND STEWS

PER SERVING
CALORIES: 183
TOTAL FAT: 7 G
SODIUM: 121 MG
CARBS: 28 G
SUGAR: 10 G
PROTEIN: 3 G

2 tablespoons coconut oil

2 pounds sweet onions (about 6), halved and cut into ¼-inch slices

1 tablespoon chopped fresh thyme or ½ teaspoon dried thyme

Juice of ½ lime

5 cups Easy Beef Bone Broth (page 268)

¼ teaspoon sea salt

1. Place a large heavy-bottom saucepan over low heat and warm the coconut oil.

2. Add the onions and thyme, stirring to coat the vegetables in oil.

3. Cover the saucepan with a lid and allow the onions to steam in their own juices until they are reduced, about 20 minutes.

4. Remove the lid from the pot and continue to caramelize the onions slowly, stirring occasionally, until they are a deep caramel color, about 90 minutes.

5. Add the lime juice and beef broth and increase the heat to medium to bring the soup to a simmer.

6. Lower the heat and simmer for 1 hour to intensify the flavor of the soup.

7. Season with salt and serve.

SIMPLE BORSCHT

▸ Serves 4

▸ Prep time: 15 minutes ▸ Cook time: 25 minutes

Borscht is a peasant dish originating and still popular in Eastern Europe, including Ukraine, Russia, Lithuania, and Poland. The recipe has many variations and can be vegetarian, thick, broth-like, smooth with cream, or chunky with meat. This recipe has a rich beet flavor that is brightened by a splash of lemon juice.

1 tablespoon extra-virgin olive oil

½ sweet onion, chopped

2 teaspoons minced fresh garlic

3 cups peeled and diced beets

1 cup shredded red cabbage

1 cup peeled and chopped carrot

4 cups Easy Beef Bone Broth (page 268)

½ teaspoon sea salt

Juice of 1 lemon

SOUPS AND STEWS

PER SERVING

CALORIES: 110

TOTAL FAT: 4 G

SODIUM: 355 MG

CARBS: 18 G

SUGAR: 12 G

PROTEIN: 3 G

1. Place a large saucepan over medium-high heat and add the olive oil.

2. Sauté the onion and garlic in the oil until the vegetables are softened, about 3 minutes.

3. Add the beets, cabbage, and carrot, and sauté the vegetables for about 3 minutes.

4. Add the beef broth and salt and bring the soup to a boil, then reduce the heat to low and simmer until the vegetables are tender, about 20 minutes.

5. Transfer the soup to a food processor or blender and pulse until the soup is smooth, or use an immersion blender right in the saucepan.

6. Stir in the lemon juice and serve.

SQUASH-PEAR SOUP

MAKE AHEAD | *KIDS' FAVORITE* | *QUICK + EASY*

▸ Serves 4

▸ Prep time: 10 minutes ▸ Cook time: 20 minutes

This dish is a thick, subtly spiced soup that is equally good on a chilly winter evening or as part of a light lunch on a sunny spring patio. Sweet, ripe pears are an important component to this soup, both for flavor and nutrition. It is important to leave the skin on the pears because it contains at least half the fruit's dietary fiber and three to four times the antioxidants as the pear flesh. Make sure you wash your pears thoroughly, even if they are organic, to remove any contaminants.

1 winter squash (about 3 pounds), peeled, seeded, and chopped

2 pears, cored and chopped

3 cups Chicken Bone Broth (page 266)

1 teaspoon ground cinnamon

½ teaspoon ground ginger

Dash ground cloves

Dash sea salt

PER SERVING

CALORIES: 121

TOTAL FAT: 0 G

SODIUM: 15 MG

CARBS: 32 G

SUGAR: 10 G

PROTEIN: 2 G

1. Place the squash, pears, and chicken broth in a large saucepan and over medium-high heat.

2. Bring the mixture to a boil and reduce the heat to low. Simmer until the squash is tender, about 20 minutes.

3. Transfer the soup to a food processor or blender and process until the soup is smooth, or use an immersion blender right in the saucepan.

4. Add the cinnamon, ginger, cloves, and salt, and pulse to combine.

5. Serve immediately.

COCONUT SEAFOOD SOUP

QUICK + EASY | GOOD FOR BATCHES

▸ Serves 4
▸ Prep time: 15 minutes ▸ Cook time: 15 minutes

You can set this chowder down on your table in about half an hour from the first onion chopped, making it the perfect choice for dinner on a busy evening or after a long workday. Try pairing the soup with a refreshing Grapefruit Salad (page 170) to round out the meal. Any mild white fish, such as halibut, can be used for this soup—or you can try a combination of fishes. The shrimp here is 21 to 25 count. Count refers to the number of individual shrimp in a pound, so the smaller the number, the bigger the shrimp.

1 tablespoon extra-virgin olive oil

1 sweet onion, chopped

½ cup sliced mushrooms

1 teaspoon minced fresh garlic

1 teaspoon grated fresh ginger

4 cups Chicken Bone Broth (page 266)

½ cup peeled and shredded carrots

3 tilapia fillets, chopped into large chunks

10 (21 to 25 count) shrimp, peeled, deveined, and each cut into 4 pieces

1 cup unsweetened organic coconut milk (for homemade, see page 258)

1 teaspoon turmeric

¼ teaspoon sea salt

½ cup shredded spinach

PER SERVING
CALORIES: 230
TOTAL FAT: 8 G
SODIUM: 243 MG
CARBS: 10 G
SUGAR: 2 G
PROTEIN: 29 G

1. Place a large stockpot over medium-high heat and add the olive oil.
2. Sauté the onion, mushrooms, garlic, and ginger until the onion is softened, about 4 minutes.
3. Add the chicken broth and carrots and bring the soup to a boil.
4. Add the fish, shrimp, coconut milk, turmeric, and salt, and reduce the heat to low. Simmer the soup until the fish is cooked through, about 6 minutes.
5. Stir in the spinach and remove the soup from the heat.
6. Serve immediately.

CABBAGE-TURKEY SOUP

MAKE AHEAD | KIDS' FAVORITE | GOOD FOR BATCHES

- ▸ Serves 4
- ▸ Prep time: 15 minutes ▸ Cook time: 50 minutes

This recipe makes a stick-to-your-ribs soup with generous portions, so don't serve it as a first course unless you are feeding teenage football players before the big game. You could make this dish after any holiday featuring a roast turkey, because it is a great way to use up leftover meat, and the turkey carcass can be thrown in a stockpot for poultry bone broth. Turkey is an excellent source of protein—more than 30 grams per 4-ounce portion—and can help regulate blood sugar levels when combined with a complex carbohydrate such as cabbage.

SOUPS AND STEWS

PER SERVING
CALORIES: 223
TOTAL FAT: 9 G
SODIUM: 154 MG
CARBS: 24 G
SUGAR: 7 G
PROTEIN: 13 G

2 tablespoons extra-virgin olive oil

1 sweet onion, chopped

2 teaspoons minced fresh garlic

6 cups shredded green cabbage (about ½ head)

2 cups peeled and diced carrots

8 cups Chicken Bone Broth (page 266)

2 bay leaves

1 cup chopped cooked turkey

¼ teaspoon sea salt

1. Place a large saucepan over medium-high heat and add the olive oil.
2. Sauté the onion and garlic until the onion is softened, about 3 minutes.
3. Add the cabbage and carrots. Cook, stirring frequently, about 4 minutes to slightly soften the cabbage.
4. Add the chicken broth and bay leaves, bring the soup to a boil, then reduce the heat and simmer until the vegetables are tender, about 35 minutes.
5. Add the turkey and salt and simmer until the turkey is heated through, about 5 minutes.
6. Remove the bay leaves and serve.

CAULIFLOWER-BACON SOUP

MAKE AHEAD | GOOD FOR BATCHES

▸ Serves 4

▸ Prep time: 10 minutes ▸ Cook time: 30 minutes

Many cauliflower soup recipes use potato and cream to create a thick texture and rich taste. This Autoimmune Paleo Diet recipe is a bit thinner, and it has a fresher cauliflower flavor. If you like a robust soup, mix up 1 tablespoon of arrowroot powder with 3 tablespoons of water to create a paste, and whisk the paste into the hot soup before adding the blanched vegetables and bacon. In the elimination phase of the diet, black pepper is usually omitted, but parsley has a subtle peppery taste that is a good substitute. (The Italian variety tends to have more flavor than the curly leaf kind.) Store fresh, washed parsley wrapped in paper towels and sealed in a plastic bag in the refrigerator for up to 1 week.

6 strips organic bacon, chopped

2 leeks, whites only, chopped

1 teaspoon minced fresh garlic

2 heads cauliflower, cut into small florets

6 cups Chicken Bone Broth (page 266)

2 tablespoons chopped fresh parsley, for garnish

1. Fry the bacon in a large saucepan over medium-high heat, stirring frequently, until it is cooked through and crispy, about 5 minutes.

2. Transfer the bacon to a paper towel–lined plate and set aside.

3. Place the saucepan back on the heat without wiping it out, add the leeks and garlic, and sauté until they are softened, about 3 minutes.

4. Add three-fourths of the cauliflower florets and all the chicken broth to the saucepan. Add a little water to cover the cauliflower if the liquid is not at least 1 inch above the vegetables.

5. Bring the soup to a boil, then reduce the heat to low and simmer until the cauliflower is tender, about 20 minutes.

6. While the soup is simmering, place a small saucepan of water on high heat and bring it to a boil. ▸

SOUPS AND STEWS

PER SERVING

CALORIES: 152

TOTAL FAT: 5 G

SODIUM: 272 MG

CARBS: 21 G

SUGAR: 5 G

PROTEIN: 6 G

Cauliflower-Bacon Soup *continued*

7. Blanch the remaining one-fourth of cauliflower until tender-crisp, about 3 minutes.

8. Drain the blanched cauliflower and set aside.

9. Transfer the soup to a food processor or blender and process until it is smooth, or use an immersion blender right in the saucepan.

10. Pour the soup back in the saucepan and add the blanched cauliflower and bacon.

11. Serve the soup garnished with fresh chopped parsley.

SOUPS AND
STEWS

VEGETABLE AND BEEF SOUP

MAKE AHEAD | KIDS' FAVORITE | GOOD FOR BATCHES

▶ Serves 4

▶ Prep time: 15 minutes ▶ Cook time: 30 minutes

This colorful soup has a double dose of rich beef flavor, from the broth and the ground beef. If you can't find very lean ground beef, you will have to scoop out and discard some of the accumulated fat after the beef is cooked in step 1. It is best to have only about 1 tablespoon of fat in the pot for sautéing the vegetables, or your soup will be greasy.

1 pound lean ground beef

3 celery stalks, diced

1 sweet onion, diced

2 teaspoons minced fresh garlic

5 cups Easy Beef Bone Broth (page 268)

2 carrots, peeled and sliced into disks

2 parsnips, peeled and diced

1 sweet potato, peeled and diced

1 cup shredded cabbage

1 tablespoon chopped fresh thyme or 1 teaspoon dried thyme

¼ teaspoon sea salt

2 tablespoons chopped fresh parsley, for garnish

SOUPS AND STEWS

PER SERVING
CALORIES: 340
TOTAL FAT: 7 G
SODIUM: 260 MG
CARBS: 30 G
SUGAR: 8 G
PROTEIN: 37 G

1. Sauté the ground beef in a medium stockpot over medium-high heat until it is cooked through, about 5 minutes.

2. Add the celery, onion, and garlic, and sauté until the vegetables are tender, about 4 minutes.

3. Add the beef broth, carrots, parsnips, and sweet potato, and bring the liquid to a simmer.

4. Reduce the heat to low and simmer the soup for 10 minutes.

5. Add the cabbage and thyme and simmer until the vegetables are tender, about 10 minutes.

6. Stir in the salt.

7. Serve the soup garnished with fresh parsley.

SAVORY LAMB STEW

MAKE AHEAD | GOOD FOR BATCHES

- ▸ Serves 4
- ▸ Prep time: 30 minutes ▸ Cook time: 2 hours, 15 minutes

The distinctly North African accents of this savory dish are a fragrant surprise. Warm spices create a broth with a full-bodied flavor that is infused into the meat when it is cooked slowly. This is a perfect recipe to double, because the finished stew freezes beautifully. Although this recipe is meant to stand alone, it can also be served over mashed cauliflower for a more substantial meal. This stew would also be nice with venison instead of lamb.

SOUPS AND STEWS

PER SERVING
CALORIES: 421
TOTAL FAT: 19 G
SODIUM: 209 MG
CARBS: 11 G
SUGAR: 3 G
PROTEIN: 49 G

2 tablespoons extra-virgin olive oil

1½ pounds lamb shoulder, trimmed of visible fat and cut into 2-inch chunks

½ sweet onion, chopped

2 teaspoons minced fresh garlic

1 teaspoon grated fresh ginger

½ teaspoon ground cinnamon

½ teaspoon turmeric

¼ teaspoon ground cloves

2 cups peeled and diced carrots

2 cups Easy Beef Bone Broth (page 268)

¼ teaspoon sea salt

2 tablespoons chopped fresh cilantro, for garnish

1. Preheat the oven to 300°F.
2. Place a large ovenproof casserole dish on the stove top over medium-high heat and add the olive oil.
3. Brown the lamb in the oil, stirring occasionally, about 4 minutes.
4. Add the onion, garlic, ginger, cinnamon, turmeric, and cloves, and sauté until the onion is softened, about 4 minutes.
5. Add the carrots, beef broth, and salt, bring the stew to a boil, then cover the container, and place it in the oven.
6. Cook the stew in the oven until the lamb is very tender, about 2 hours.
7. Remove the stew from the oven and serve it hot, garnished with cilantro.

CREAMY CHICKEN STEW WITH APPLE

MAKE AHEAD | GOOD FOR BATCHES

▸ Makes 6 servings

▸ Prep time: 15 minutes ▸ Cook time: 45 minutes

This is the perfect meal when you are coming in rosy cheeked from activities outside or times you want to make a huge pot to take to a family potluck. If you can't find fresh tarragon, do not substitute dried products because the flavor is not the same. Try thyme instead in the same amount if tarragon is not available.

2 teaspoons olive oil

2 pounds boneless, skinless chicken breasts, cut into 1-inch chunks

1 sweet onion, chopped

1 celery stalk, sliced

1 teaspoon minced fresh garlic

½ pound carrots (about 5), diced

½ pound parsnips (about 5), diced

1 sweet potato, diced

1 apple, peeled, cored, and diced

1 can unsweetened organic coconut milk

1 cup Chicken Bone Broth (page 266)

1 teaspoon sea salt

2 tablespoons chopped fresh tarragon

SOUPS AND STEWS

PER SERVING
CALORIES: 484
TOTAL FAT: 22G
SODIUM: 490MG
CARBS: 24G
SUGARS: 10G
PROTEIN: 46G

1. Place a large heavy-bottom pan over medium high heat and add the olive oil.

2. Brown the chicken chunks in batches and set them aside on a plate.

3. Add the onion, celery, and garlic to the skillet and sauté until lightly browned, about five minutes.

4. Add the carrots, parsnip, sweet potato, apple, coconut milk, and chicken broth to the skillet with the reserved chicken.

5. Stir to combine and bring the stew to a boil.

6. Reduce the heat to low and simmer the stew until the chicken is tender and cooked through and the vegetables are soft, about 40 minutes.

7. Season with salt and serve topped with tarragon.

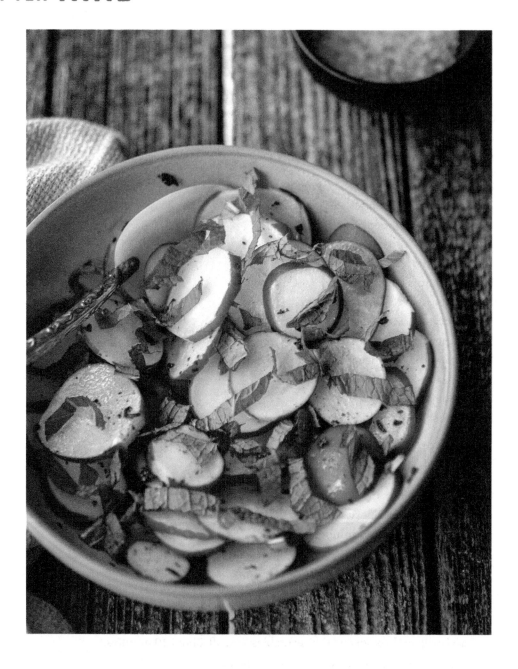

SALADS

GRILLED ZUCCHINI SALAD

GOOD FOR BATCHES

▸ Serves 4

▸ Prep time: 15 minutes, plus 30 minutes to cool ▸ Cook time: 8 minutes

The best zucchini for this attractive salad are medium to smaller squash, because the large ones can be fibrous and even a little bitter. Mixing yellow and green zucchini can create a truly lovely presentation if you take the time to arrange your slices and onion in concentric circles on a serving plate. You can even replace the plain balsamic vinegar with a drizzle of rich Balsamic Reduction (page 103) to create a visual and flavorful impact.

2 pounds zucchini (about 6), cut into ¼-inch-thick slices

½ sweet onion, sliced

¼ cup extra-virgin olive oil

2 tablespoons gluten-free balsamic vinegar

¼ teaspoon sea salt

½ cup shredded fresh basil

1. Place the zucchini and onion slices in a medium bowl and toss with the olive oil.

2. Preheat a barbecue to medium heat.

3. Grill the zucchini and onion until tender and lightly charred, turning once, about 4 minutes per side.

4. If you do not have a barbecue, preheat the oven to 450°F, and spread the vegetables on a baking tray. Roast them in the oven, turning once, until they are lightly browned and tender, about 10 minutes total.

5. Transfer the grilled or roasted vegetables to a bowl and let them cool for about 30 minutes.

6. Add the balsamic vinegar, salt, and basil, and toss to combine before serving.

SALADS

PER SERVING

CALORIES: 152

TOTAL FAT: 13 G

SODIUM: 127 MG

CARBS: 9 G

SUGAR: 4 G

PROTEIN: 3 G

NECTARINE-CUCUMBER SALAD

MAKE AHEAD | KIDS' FAVORITE | QUICK+EASY | GOOD FOR BATCHES

- ▸ Serves 4
- ▸ Prep time: 15 minutes

Nectarines are often overlooked when sitting next to their more flagrantly beautiful fuzzy counterpart, peaches. Nectarines provide twice the vitamin A as well as more vitamin C and potassium than peaches. To get the best flavor, buy organic nectarines and let them ripen at room temperature for a few days rather than placing them in the refrigerator.

2 nectarines, pitted and diced into ½-inch chunks

2 English cucumbers, diced into ½-inch chunks

1 cup halved snap peas

½ cup chopped fresh mint

1 tablespoon freshly squeezed lemon juice

1. Mix the nectarines, cucumber, snap peas, mint, and lemon juice in a large bowl until well combined.

2. Serve immediately.

SALADS

PER SERVING
CALORIES: 69
TOTAL FAT: 1 G
SODIUM: 7 MG
CARBS: 16 G
SUGAR: 6 G
PROTEIN: 3 G

JICAMA-FENNEL SALAD

▸ Serves 4

▸ Prep time: 20 minutes

The unusual crispness of this salad will be the first thing you notice, before the fragrance of basil and licorice-like fennel take over. Jicama and fennel are both juicy, crunchy vegetables, so the combination creates a salad that almost quenches your thirst. When choosing the jicama for this dish, try to get small ones, about 5 inches in diameter, because they are sweeter than the larger vegetables.

SALADS

PER SERVING
CALORIES: 232
TOTAL FAT: 14 G
SODIUM: 51 MG
CARBS: 26 G
SUGAR: 8 G
PROTEIN: 3 G

FOR THE DRESSING
4 tablespoons extra-virgin olive oil
2 tablespoons apple cider vinegar
1 tablespoon chopped fresh basil

FOR THE SALAD
1 fennel bulb, thinly sliced
1 jicama, peeled and diced
1 apple, cored and diced
1 tablespoon freshly squeezed lemon juice
2 cups shredded spinach

TO MAKE THE DRESSING

Whisk the olive oil, apple cider vinegar, and basil in a small bowl until well combined, and set aside.

TO MAKE THE SALAD

1. Toss the fennel, jicama, apple, and lemon juice in a large bowl until well combined.

2. Add the spinach and dressing, and toss to combine.

3. Serve immediately.

FRUITED SWEET POTATO SALAD

▸ Serves 4

▸ Prep time: 15 minutes

Potato salad is often mayonnaise-soaked chunks of starchy white potato with a smattering of onion or grated hard-boiled egg. The colors, different textures, and glorious array of individual flavors of this sweet potato creation will change your opinion of boring potato salad forever. Sweet potatoes are an almost unparalleled source of beta-carotene and are high in vitamins A, B_6 and C as well as manganese and copper.

2 pounds cooked sweet potatoes (about 5 large), cut into ½-inch chunks

½ cup chopped sweet onion

1 apple, cored and diced

½ cup dried cranberries

2 tablespoons freshly squeezed lemon juice

Pinch sea salt

1. Toss the sweet potato, onion, apple, cranberries, and lemon juice in a large bowl until well combined.

2. Season the salad with salt and serve.

SALADS

PER SERVING

CALORIES: 305

TOTAL FAT: 1 G

SODIUM: 45 MG

CARBS: 72 G

SUGAR: 7 G

PROTEIN: 4 G

GRAPEFRUIT SALAD

QUICK+EASY

- ▸ Serves 4
- ▸ Prep time: 15 minutes

Red grapefruits are a splendid choice for fresh fruit when most other fruit is not in season. Grapefruits are available year-round, but they are in season through the winter and early spring, so try to use them when they're at their best. You can use white grapefruits in this recipe, but the red variety is a little sweeter and provides the added benefit of the phytonutrient lycopene. Lycopene can help lower the risk of some cancers, such as prostate cancer, and promote a healthy cardiovascular system.

FOR THE DRESSING

½ cup extra-virgin olive oil

2 tablespoons apple cider vinegar

1 tablespoon local organic honey

1 teaspoon freshly squeezed lemon juice

Pinch sea salt

FOR THE SALAD

3 cups spinach

2 red grapefruits, peeled, sectioned, and chopped

¼ cup dried cranberries

TO MAKE THE DRESSING

Whisk the olive oil, vinegar, honey, lemon juice, and salt in a small bowl until well combined, and set aside.

TO MAKE THE SALAD

1. Mix the spinach, grapefruits, and cranberries in a large bowl until well combined.

2. Add the dressing and toss to combine.

3. Serve immediately.

SALADS

PER SERVING
CALORIES: 268
TOTAL FAT: 25 G
SODIUM: 77 MG
CARBS: 13 G
SUGAR: 9 G
PROTEIN: 1 G

MINTED RADISH SALAD

MAKE AHEAD | KIDS' FAVORITE | QUICK+EASY | GOOD FOR BATCHES

▸ Serves 4
▸ Prep time: 20 minutes, plus 30 minutes to marinate

Simple, fresh flavors and very few ingredients create a perfect salad for a backyard barbecue or a picnic on a sunny day in the park. Radish is a rich source of dietary fiber, vitamin C, potassium, calcium, and magnesium. This pungent tasting vegetable has a cooling effect on the body and in Eastern and Ayurvedic healing is used purge toxins and free radicals from the body.

3 pounds small red radishes, sliced
1 cup finely shredded fresh mint
Juice of 1 lemon
¼ teaspoon sea salt

1. Mix the sliced radish, mint, lemon juice, and salt in a large bowl until well combined.

2. Place the salad in the refrigerator for at least 30 minutes so the flavors combine before serving.

SALADS

PER SERVING
CALORIES 67
TOTAL FAT: 0 G
SODIUM: 257 MG
CARBS: 14 G
SUGAR: 7 G
PROTEIN: 3 G

WALDORF SALAD

QUICK + EASY

▶ Serves 4

▶ Prep time: 15 minutes, plus 15 minutes to chill

The apples need to be sweet and still crisp to create the perfect foil for the other ingredients. Apples sold in the summer have been stored almost a full year in climate-controlled refrigeration units, and if the apples were originally picked too late, the natural starches turn to sugar, creating an unpleasant, mealy texture. When in doubt, ask your local grocer to cut open one of the apples so you can sample it. The chicken in this recipe does not have to come from the breast meat; dark meat from the thighs or drumsticks is very tasty. If you have roasted chicken for dinner, this salad is a delicious way to use up leftovers the next day for lunch.

SALADS

PER SERVING
CALORIES: 282
TOTAL FAT: 8 G
SODIUM: 146 MG
CARBS: 19 G
SUGAR: 14 G
PROTEIN: 33 G

2 apples, cored and chopped

¼ cup freshly squeezed lemon juice

1 pound cooked boneless, skinless chicken, chopped

8 celery stalks, sliced

3 cups shredded spinach

1 cup halved green grapes

1. Mix the apples and lemon juice in a large bowl until the apple chunks are well coated.

2. Add the chicken, celery, spinach, and grapes, and toss until well combined.

3. Place the salad in the refrigerator to chill for about 15 minutes before serving.

ROASTED SWEET POTATO SALAD

GOOD FOR BATCHES

▸ Serves 4

▸ Prep time: 10 minutes ▸ Cook time: 50 minutes

This warm, crispy, bacon-studded salad is the ideal comfort food. It's like being wrapped in a cozy blanket on a chilly winter evening. You can boil or steam your potatoes instead of cooking them in the oven, but roasting adds an extra element of mellow sweetness to this dish. Try pairing the salad with juicy Lamb Sliders (page 224) for a lovely, filling dinner.

4 large sweet potatoes (about 2 pounds), peeled and diced into ½-inch chunks
8 slices organic bacon, chopped
1 sweet onion, chopped
½ cup apple cider vinegar

SALADS

PER SERVING
CALORIES: 366
TOTAL FAT: 7 G
SODIUM: 292 MG
CARBS: 66 G
SUGAR: 3 G
PROTEIN: 8 G

1. Preheat the oven to 350°F.

2. Line a baking sheet with parchment paper and set aside.

3. Place the sweet potatoes in a large bowl and set aside.

4. Place a medium skillet over medium-high heat and cook the bacon until it is crispy, about 5 minutes.

5. Transfer the bacon to a paper towel–lined plate.

6. Add 1 tablespoon of bacon fat to the sweet potatoes and reserve the rest of the fat for another recipe.

7. Toss the potatoes with the fat and transfer them to the baking tray.

8. Roast the sweet potatoes until they are golden and crispy, about 45 minutes. Add the chopped onion to the baking tray for the last 15 minutes of cooking time.

9. Transfer the sweet potato mixture to a large bowl, add the apple cider vinegar and cooked bacon, and toss to combine.

10. Serve warm.

SALMON AND BEET SALAD

QUICK + EASY

- ▸ Serves 4
- ▸ Prep time: 15 minutes

Salmon is a rich source of omega-3 fatty acids, which are important because they can help decrease inflammation in the joints, support nerve and brain health, and reduce the risk of cardiovascular disease. This gorgeous salad can be topped with either fresh or BPA-free canned salmon. Oranges add a gorgeous color and satisfying, subtle sweetness to the salad. Oranges are a stellar source of vitamin C, which can help support a healthy immune system and reduce the risk of cardiovascular disease. Oranges are also a rich source of fiber, which can help stabilize blood sugar and support the digestive system.

SALADS

PER SERVING
CALORIES: 220
TOTAL FAT: 17 G
SODIUM: 128 MG
CARBS: 10 G
SUGAR: 6 G
PROTEIN: 10 G

FOR THE DRESSING
4 tablespoons extra-virgin olive oil
1 tablespoon apple cider vinegar
1 teaspoon orange zest
Pinch sea salt

FOR THE SALAD
4 cups spinach
½ red onion, halved and thinly sliced
½ large orange, peeled and chopped
1 cup peeled and diced cooked beets
6 ounces cooked salmon, flaked

TO MAKE THE DRESSING

Whisk the olive oil, vinegar, orange zest, and salt in a small bowl until well combined, and set aside.

TO MAKE THE SALAD

1. Toss the spinach, onion, orange, and beets in a large bowl until well combined.

2. Add the dressing to the salad and toss lightly to combine.

3. Top the salad with the salmon and serve.

TRADITIONAL COLESLAW

MAKE AHEAD | KIDS' FAVORITE | QUICK+EASY | GOOD FOR BATCHES

▸ Serves 4

▸ Prep time: 20 minutes, plus 1 hour to marinate

This recipe makes full-size portions of coleslaw rather than a meager side dish. Leaving out the mayonnaise in the dressing allows the crisp, pungent flavor of the cabbage and sweet, earthy carrot to shine through. You can also add about ½ cup of thinly sliced onion to this slaw for a more intense flavor. This coleslaw is even better if you leave it in the refrigerator overnight so the flavors can blend and it can pickle slightly. Make it ahead of time rather than eating it right away, or double the recipe so you'll have leftovers.

FOR THE DRESSING

¼ cup extra-virgin olive oil

¼ cup apple cider vinegar

1 tablespoon local organic honey

¼ teaspoon garlic powder

Pinch sea salt

FOR THE SALAD

3 cups shredded green cabbage (¼ head)

3 cups shredded red cabbage (¼ head)

2 cups peeled and shredded carrots

SALADS

PER SERVING

CALORIES: 178

TOTAL FAT: 12 G

SODIUM: 54 MG

CARBS: 16 G

SUGAR: 10 G

PROTEIN: 2 G

TO MAKE THE DRESSING

Whisk the olive oil, vinegar, honey, garlic powder, and salt in a small bowl until well combined, and set aside.

TO MAKE THE SALAD

1. Toss the green and red cabbage and carrots in a large bowl until well combined.

2. Add the dressing and toss to combine.

3. Let the salad stand at least 1 hour before serving.

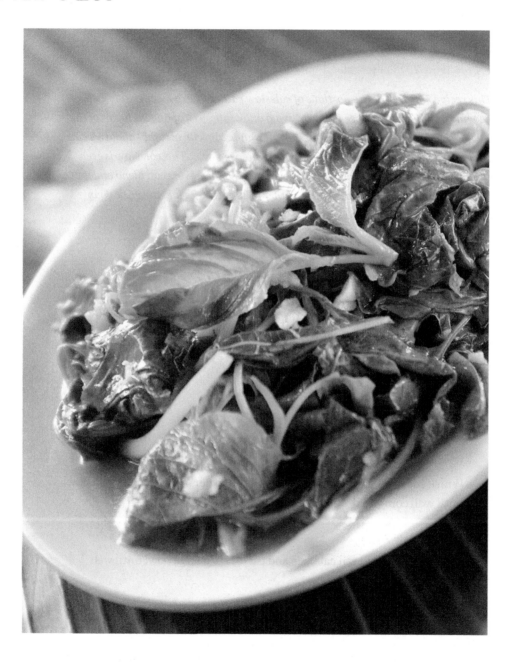

SIDE DISHES

MASHED CAULIFLOWER

KIDS' FAVORITE | QUICK + EASY | GOOD FOR BATCHES

▶ Serves 4

▶ Prep time: 10 minutes ▶ Cook time: 10 minutes

This substitute for mashed potatoes does not taste exactly like the original, but you might be surprised to find it is just as good, and extra smooth and creamy. If you want your mashed cauliflower to have a little more texture, try using a potato masher instead of the food processor. The trick to mashed cauliflower is to control the water content, so steaming your florets is probably the best cooking choice if you have a steamer. If not, supervise the blanching process carefully and add the coconut milk in increments to get the perfect texture.

1 head cauliflower (about 3 pounds), cut into small florets
1 teaspoon minced fresh garlic
½ cup unsweetened organic coconut milk (for homemade, see page 258)
¼ teaspoon sea salt

1. Place a large pot of water on high heat and bring to a boil.

2. Blanch the cauliflower until it is tender but not waterlogged, about 5 minutes.

3. Drain the cauliflower thoroughly and transfer it to a food processor.

4. Place the garlic and coconut milk in a small saucepan over medium-high heat and cook for about 2 minutes. Do not boil.

5. Add the garlic milk to the cauliflower and purée until it is creamy and thick, about 2 minutes. Alternately, mash the cauliflower and garlic milk by hand in a large bowl, using a potato masher.

6. Transfer the mashed cauliflower to a bowl and season with salt.

7. Serve immediately.

SIDE DISHES

PER SERVING
CALORIES: 123
TOTAL FAT: 7 G
SODIUM: 122 MG
CARBS: 13 G
SUGAR: 6 G
PROTEIN: 5 G

BAKED PARSNIP AND SWEET POTATO FRIES

FODMAP-FREE | KIDS' FAVORITE | GOOD FOR BATCHES

▸ Serves 4

▸ Prep time: 10 minutes ▸ Cook time: 35 minutes

Parsnip looks a little like a cream-colored carrot but has a distinct taste all its own, which gets sweeter when roasted. Parsnips are low in calories and high in potassium, folic acid, and fiber. They can help reduce the risk of dementia and cardiovascular disease and help regulate blood sugar.

3 parsnips, peeled and cut into ½-inch-wide sticks

1 sweet potato, peeled and cut into ½-inch-wide sticks

¼ cup extra-virgin olive oil

¼ teaspoon sea salt

1. Preheat the oven to 450°F.

2. Line a baking sheet with parchment paper and set aside.

3. Place the parsnips, sweet potato, olive oil, and salt in a large bowl and toss to combine.

4. Transfer the fries to the baking sheet and spread them out evenly, with no overlap.

5. Bake the fries until they are golden and crispy, turning them a few times, about 35 minutes total.

6. Serve immediately.

SIDE DISHES

PER SERVING

CALORIES: 208

TOTAL FAT: 13 G

SODIUM: 122 MG

CARBS: 23 G

SUGAR: 7 G

PROTEIN: 2 G

SPICED BROCCOLI

► Serves 4

► Prep time: 10 minutes ► Cook time: 10 minutes

Fresh ginger adds a pleasing heat and Asian flavor to this sautéed broccoli and onion. Ginger has been used medicinally for centuries for digestive system upsets such as nausea and indigestion. Ginger also fights free radicals in the body, and its anti-inflammatory properties can help reduce the pain associated with arthritis.

1 tablespoon coconut oil

½ cup thinly sliced sweet onion

1 teaspoon grated fresh ginger

½ teaspoon minced fresh garlic

2 broccoli heads, cut into small florets

2 tablespoons water

SIDE DISHES

PER SERVING
CALORIES 98
TOTAL FAT: 4 G
SODIUM: 130 MG
CARBS: 13 G
SUGAR: 4 G
PROTEIN: 5 G

1. Place a large skillet over medium-high heat and add the coconut oil.

2. Sauté the onion, ginger, and garlic until softened, about 3 minutes.

3. Add the broccoli and water and sauté until the broccoli is tender, about 5 minutes.

4. Serve immediately.

SAUTÉED FENNEL AND RADICCHIO WITH APPLE

QUICK + EASY

- ▶ Serves 4
- ▶ Prep time: 10 minutes ▶ Cook time: 10 minutes

Radicchio is an undeniable pretty leafy vegetable with white-veined, deep red leaves. Its assertive bitter taste can be a bit of a shock but makes it a delicious choice to sauté with savory ingredients and strong spices. The fennel and apple in this recipe mellow the taste of the radicchio, so if you are unfamiliar with radicchio, this recipe is a good place to start. Radicchio is high in antioxidants, such as zeaxanthin and lutein, that can protect against age-related macular disease. It is also a rich source of vitamin K, which may reduce the risk and effects of Alzheimer's disease.

1 tablespoon extra-virgin olive oil
1 teaspoon minced fresh garlic
1 small fennel bulb, thinly sliced
1 small head radicchio, thinly sliced
1 apple, peeled, cored, and diced
Juice of ½ lemon
¼ teaspoon sea salt

SIDE DISHES

PER SERVING
CALORIES 78
TOTAL FAT: 4 G
SODIUM: 153 MG
CARBS: 12 G
SUGAR: 5 G
PROTEIN: 1 G

1. Place a large skillet over medium heat and add the olive oil.
2. When the oil is hot, add the garlic and sauté until fragrant, about 2 minutes.
3. Add the fennel and sauté until the vegetable softens, about 4 minutes.
4. Add the radicchio and sauté until it starts to wilt, about 2 minutes.
5. Remove the skillet from the heat and stir in the apple, lemon juice, and salt before serving.

CARROT RIBBONS WITH PARSLEY

KIDS' FAVORITE | QUICK + EASY

▸ Serves 4

▸ Prep time: 15 minutes ▸ Cook time: 10 minutes

The secret to making an attractive ribbon salad is to be very gentle with the carrot "noodles" while sautéing. The ribbons will break if you toss them around too much, either when they are still raw or softened. Carrots are known for their high beta-carotene content, but they are also a good source of other disease-fighting antioxidants, such as hydroxycinnamic acids and anthocyanins. These antioxidants mean carrots can have a significant positive impact on general good health.

SIDE DISHES

1 teaspoon extra-virgin olive oil

1 teaspoon minced fresh garlic

1½ pounds carrots (6 or 7), peeled and cut into long ribbons
      with a vegetable peeler

2 tablespoons chopped fresh parsley, for garnish

PER SERVING
CALORIES: 105
TOTAL FAT: 1 G
SODIUM: 157 MG
CARBS: 23 G
SUGAR: 11 G
PROTEIN: 2 G

1. Place a large skillet over medium heat and add the olive oil.

2. Add the garlic and sauté until it is fragrant, about 2 minutes.

3. Add the carrot ribbons and sauté carefully until the carrots are tender-crisp, about 5 minutes.

4. Remove the skillet from the heat and serve garnished with parsley.

STIR-FRIED BRUSSELS SPROUTS

QUICK + EASY

- ▶ Serves 4
- ▶ Prep time: 15 minutes ▶ Cook time: 15 minutes

Brussels sprouts look like mini cabbages, and these tiny cruciferous vegetables are packed with nutrients. One cup of Brussels sprouts contains almost 250 percent of the recommended daily allowance (RDA) of vitamin K and more than 125 percent of the RDA of vitamin C. This means Brussels sprouts are powerful disease fighters and can help detoxify the body.

1 teaspoon extra-virgin olive oil
½ cup thinly sliced sweet onion
1 teaspoon minced fresh garlic
1 teaspoon grated fresh ginger
2 pounds Brussels sprouts, halved
1 tablespoon local organic honey
¼ teaspoon sea salt

1. Place a large skillet over medium heat and add the olive oil.

2. Sauté the onion, garlic, and ginger until the onion is softened, about 3 minutes.

3. Add the Brussels sprouts and sauté until they are tender-crisp, about 8 minutes.

4. Remove the skillet from heat, add the honey and salt, and stir to combine.

5. Serve immediately.

SIDE DISHES

PER SERVING
CALORIES: 133
TOTAL FAT: 2 G
SODIUM: 174 MG
CARBS: 27 G
SUGAR: 10 G
PROTEIN: 8 G

ROASTED THYME SWEET POTATOES

▶ Serves 4

▶ Prep time: 10 minutes ▶ Cook time: 30 minutes

Herbs are usually thought of in culinary terms, but for centuries they have also been regarded as potent medicines. Many modern medications are derived from herbs. Thyme is historically a treatment for respiratory problems such as congestion and cough, but it is also surprisingly nutrient-dense for such a delicate plant. Thyme is a wonderful source of vitamins A and C as well as a good source of copper, iron, and fiber.

SIDE DISHES

4 sweet potatoes, peeled and cut into 1½-inch chunks

2 tablespoons chopped fresh thyme

3 teaspoons extra-virgin olive oil

1 teaspoon minced fresh garlic

⅛ teaspoon sea salt

PER SERVING

CALORIES: 300

TOTAL FAT: 4 G

SODIUM: 64 MG

CARBS: 64 G

SUGAR: 1 G

PROTEIN: 4 G

1. Preheat the oven to 400°F.

2. Line a baking sheet with parchment paper and set aside.

3. Place the sweet potato chunks, thyme, olive oil, garlic, and salt in a medium bowl and toss until well combined.

4. Transfer the potato mixture to the baking sheet and spread it out in a single layer.

5. Roast the potato mixture until the potatoes are crispy and golden, turning at least twice, about 30 minutes.

6. Serve immediately.

MIXED SAUTÉED VEGETABLES

KIDS' FAVORITE | QUICK+EASY

▸ Serves 4

▸ Prep time: 10 minutes ▸ Cook time: 10 minutes

The mix of vegetables in this dish can be changed depending on what you have in your refrigerator or your personal taste. The technique used to create perfect tender vegetables is half sautéing and half steaming. Adding water by tablespoons to the hot skillet creates a humid cooking environment that speeds the cooking process and keeps the vegetables from browning.

1 teaspoon extra-virgin olive oil

2 cups broccoli florets

2 cups cauliflower florets

2 tablespoons water

1 cup peeled and sliced carrots

1 cup asparagus spears, cut into 3-inch pieces

Pinch sea salt

1. Place a large skillet over medium heat and add the olive oil.

2. Sauté the broccoli, cauliflower, and 1 tablespoon of water for 4 minutes.

3. Add the carrots and the remaining 1 tablespoon of water, and sauté until the carrots are tender-crisp, about 2 minutes.

4. Add the asparagus and sauté until the asparagus is tender-crisp, about 1 minute.

5. Season the vegetables with salt before serving.

SIDE DISHES

PER SERVING

CALORIES 69

TOTAL FAT: 1 G

SODIUM: 298 MG

CARBS: 12 G

SUGAR: 5 G

PROTEIN: 4 G

WILTED GREENS

▸ Serves 4

▸ Prep time: 10 minutes ▸ Cook time: 5 minutes

This dish is the simplest form of wilted greens. The splash of vinegar brightens the dish and makes your taste buds take notice. You can also use freshly squeezed lemon juice to create this intensifying effect. This dish would make a nice accompaniment for a salmon or halibut main course. The greens have an assertive taste that would not be overpowered by the fish, and you could place the fillets right on a bed of greens for an elegant presentation. Good choices of mixed greens include arugula, chard, kale, and spinach.

SIDE DISHES

PER SERVING
CALORIES: 210
TOTAL FAT: 7 G
SODIUM: 140 MG
CARBS: 30 G
SUGAR: 7 G
PROTEIN: 7 G

2 tablespoons extra-virgin olive oil

1 teaspoon chopped fresh garlic

2 pounds mixed leafy greens, coarse stems removed and leaves chopped

2 tablespoons apple cider vinegar

¼ teaspoon salt

1. Place a large skillet over medium-high heat and add the olive oil.

2. Add the garlic and saute for one minute.

3. Add the greens and vinegar to the skillet and use tongs to toss the greens continuously until they are wilted, about 5 minutes.

4. Season the greens with salt before serving.

SAUTÉED GARLICKY MUSHROOMS

▸ Serves 4

▸ Prep time: 3 minutes ▸ Cook time: 10 minutes

If you are having grilled beef or venison for dinner, these tender mushrooms are a superlative topping. Mushrooms aren't just delicious; they also provide impressive support to the immune system. Mushrooms help balance the activity of white blood cells in the body, which may help prevent many diseases such as cardiovascular disease, cancer, and arthritis.

1 tablespoon extra-virgin olive oil
2 pounds button mushrooms, halved
1 teaspoon minced fresh garlic
1 tablespoon gluten-free balsamic vinegar
Pinch sea salt

1. Place a large skillet over medium-high heat and add the olive oil.
2. Sauté the mushrooms, stirring frequently, until they are lightly browned and tender, about 6 minutes.
3. Add the garlic and sauté for 2 minutes.
4. Remove the skillet from the heat, add the vinegar, and toss to combine.
5. Season the mushrooms with salt before serving.

SIDE DISHES

PER SERVING
CALORIES 60
TOTAL FAT: 4 G
SODIUM: 124 MG
CARBS: 5 G
SUGAR: 3 G
PROTEIN: 4 G

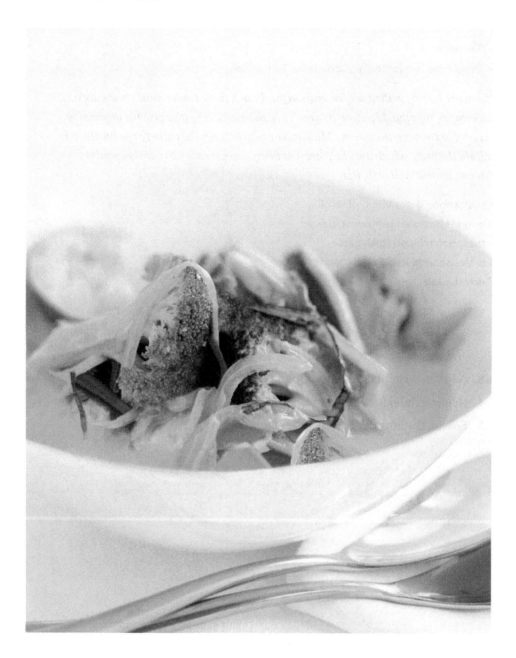

VEGETARIAN DINNERS

STIR-FRIED VEGETABLES WITH CAULIFLOWER "RICE"

KIDS' FAVORITE | QUICK + EASY

▸ Serves 4

▸ Prep time: 15 minutes ▸ Cook time: 15 minutes

Finely chopped cauliflower might sound like a strange base for this dish, but it mimics rice quite well. Cauliflower has many nutritional benefits, as do all the cruciferous vegetables, and is an anti-inflammatory and an antioxidant. Cauliflower is high in vitamins C and K as well as many B vitamins and omega-3 essential fatty acids. It may help reduce the risk of cancer and cardiovascular disease, and it supports healthy brain function and effective digestion.

VEGETARIAN DINNERS

PER SERVING
CALORIES: 110
TOTAL FAT: 4 G
SODIUM: 125 MG
CARBS: 17 G
SUGAR: 6 G
PROTEIN: 4 G

4 cups chopped cauliflower

3 teaspoons extra-virgin olive oil

3 teaspoons minced fresh garlic

¼ cup water

Pinch sea salt

1 cup sliced red onion

1 tablespoon grated fresh ginger

2 cups broccoli florets

1 cup peeled and sliced carrots

1 cup halved snap peas

Juice of ½ lemon

2 tablespoons chopped fresh cilantro, for garnish

1. Place the cauliflower in a food processor and pulse until it is finely chopped, or use a chef's knife or a cleaver to chop the cauliflower until it resembles fine crumbs.

2. Place a large skillet over medium heat and add 1 teaspoon of olive oil.

3. Sauté 1 teaspoon of garlic until it is fragrant and softened, about 2 minutes.

4. Add the cauliflower, water, and salt to the skillet, cover, and steam the cauliflower until it is tender-crisp, about 2 minutes.

5. Transfer the cauliflower to a bowl and cover. Set aside.

6. Wipe out the skillet and add the remaining 2 teaspoons of olive oil. Set the skillet over medium-high heat.

7. Add the remaining 2 teaspoons of garlic, plus the onion and ginger, and sauté until the onion is softened, about 3 minutes.

8. Add the broccoli florets, carrots, and snap peas, and sauté until tender, about 6 minutes.

9. Remove the vegetables from the heat and add the lemon juice.

10. Serve the vegetables over the cauliflower, garnished with the cilantro.

VEGETARIAN DINNERS

RADISH AND JICAMA TABBOULEH

FODMAP-FREE | MAKE AHEAD | QUICK+EASY

▸ Serves 4

▸ Prep time: 20 minutes, plus 1 hour to chill

Tabbouleh is a North African dish usually made with bulgur wheat and finely chopped herbs and vegetables. This recipe omits the bulgur and uses starchy jicama instead to provide the foundation. Radishes add a distinct heat to the dish as well as vitamin B_6, iron, copper, and calcium. A food processor makes this dish a snap to prepare, but if you do not have this handy kitchen appliance, you can use a good knife to chop everything up finely. Chop the jicama, radishes, and carrots as uniformly as possible for the nicest presentation.

VEGETARIAN DINNERS

PER SERVING
CALORIES: 287
TOTAL FAT: 13 G
SODIUM: 123 MG
CARBS: 41 G
SUGAR: 9 G
PROTEIN: 4 G

FOR THE DRESSING

¼ cup extra-virgin olive oil

2 tablespoons apple cider vinegar

Juice and zest of ½ lemon

1 tablespoon minced mint

Pinch sea salt

FOR THE SALAD

9 radishes, tops and bottoms trimmed off

4 carrots, peeled and coarsely chopped

2 jicamas, peeled and chopped coarsely

2 English cucumbers, finely chopped

½ cup chopped fresh parsley

TO MAKE THE DRESSING

Whisk the olive oil, vinegar, lemon juice and zest, mint, and salt until well combined.

TO MAKE THE SALAD

1. Place half the radishes, carrots, and jicama in a food processor and pulse until the vegetables are finely chopped.

2. Transfer the chopped vegetables to a large bowl and repeat with the remaining vegetables. Alternately, chop all the vegetables into even, small chunks on a cutting board, then transfer them to a large bowl.

3. Add the cucumbers, dressing, and parsley and stir until well combined.

4. Chill the tabbouleh for at least 1 hour before serving.

VEGETARIAN DINNERS

VEGETABLE HASH

QUICK + EASY

▸ Serves 4
▸ Prep time: 15 minutes ▸ Cook time: 15 minutes

Hash is usually made from chopped meat, onions, and vegetables and is served most often as a breakfast dish side. This recipe is for a heartier main-meal dish spooned over creamy mashed cauliflower. The name of this dish comes from the French verb hacher, *meaning* to chop—*even though hash is not necessarily something you would see on a French restaurant menu.*

4 cups Mashed Cauliflower (page 178)

1 teaspoon extra-virgin olive oil

1 cup chopped sweet onion

2 teaspoons minced fresh garlic

2 zucchini, diced

3 cups shredded spinach

1 cup peeled, pitted, and diced avocado

1 teaspoon chopped fresh thyme

1. Warm the mashed cauliflower in a saucepan over low heat until heated through, about 5 minutes. Cover and set aside.

2. Place a large skillet over medium-high heat and add the olive oil.

3. Sauté the onion and garlic until the onion is softened, about 3 minutes.

4. Add the zucchini and sauté for 4 minutes.

5. Add the spinach and sauté for 2 minutes.

6. Serve the hash over the mashed cauliflower, topped with the diced avocado and thyme.

VEGETARIAN DINNERS

PER SERVING
CALORIES: 149
TOTAL FAT: 9 G
SODIUM: 330 MG
CARBS: 16 G
SUGAR: 6 G
PROTEIN: 5 G

THE AUTOIMMUNE PALEO COOKBOOK AND ACTION PLAN

SWEET POTATO COLCANNON

KIDS' FAVORITE

- ▸ Serves 4
- ▸ Prep time: 10 minutes ▸ Cook time: 25 minutes

This centuries-old Irish dish uses tender sautéed cabbage combined with sweet potato instead of the traditional white potato. If you'd like, you can fry up three or four strips of bacon, chop it up, and mix it with the rest of the ingredients. The bacon fat can also be used to sauté the onion, garlic, and cabbage.

2 tablespoons extra-virgin olive oil
½ sweet onion, thinly sliced
1 teaspoon minced fresh garlic
4 cups finely shredded cabbage
Pinch sea salt
4 cups mashed cooked sweet potato
½ cup unsweetened organic coconut milk (for homemade, see page 258)
½ cup chopped fresh parsley

1. Place a large skillet over medium-high heat and add the olive oil.

2. Sauté the onion and garlic until the onion is softened, about 3 minutes.

3. Add the cabbage and sauté until the cabbage is tender, about 10 minutes.

4. Season the cabbage with salt and stir in the mashed sweet potato, coconut milk, and parsley until well combined.

5. Continue to warm the sweet potato mixture until it is heated through, about 10 minutes.

6. Serve immediately.

VEGETARIAN DINNERS

PER SERVING
CALORIES: 274
TOTAL FAT: 14 G
SODIUM: 120 MG
CARBS: 35 G
SUGAR: 10 G
PROTEIN: 5 G

ROASTED ACORN SQUASH AND BRUSSELS SPROUTS

GOOD FOR BATCHES

▸ Serves 4

▸ Prep time: 10 minutes ▸ Cook time: 30 minutes

The combination of sweet, buttery squash and pungent, slightly crisp Brussels sprouts works beautifully. Acorn squash is one of those vegetables that most people buy based on size; because it is so hard, it is difficult to tell if it is ripe and ready to cook. Try to pick a squash that is heavy for its size and has more green than orange on the skin. A light squash with an uneven balance of orange can mean an older squash that will be stringy and dry. Substitute butternut squash, if you'd like.

PER SERVING
CALORIES: 140
TOTAL FAT: 4 G
SODIUM: 154 MG
CARBS: 25 G
SUGAR: 4 G
PROTEIN: 6 G

1 acorn squash (about 2 pounds), peeled, halved, seeded, and cut into ½-inch slices

6 cups halved Brussels sprouts

½ cup sliced sweet onion

2 tablespoons fresh thyme or 1 tablespoon dried thyme

1 tablespoon extra-virgin olive oil

¼ teaspoon sea salt

1. Preheat the oven to 400°F.

2. Line a baking sheet with parchment paper and set aside.

3. Toss the squash, Brussels sprouts, onion, thyme, olive oil, and salt in a large bowl until well combined.

4. Spread the squash mixture evenly on the baking sheet and roast it until the vegetables are lightly browned and tender, about 30 minutes. Stir the vegetables at least twice while they cook so that all the sides are browned evenly.

5. Serve immediately.

LIME-COCONUT ZUCCHINI NOODLES WITH AVOCADO

FODMAP-FREE | QUICK+EASY

- ▸ Serves 4
- ▸ Prep time: 15 minutes, plus 10 minutes to marinate

Zucchini noodles are a staple for many raw food enthusiasts and vegans, because the soft texture of the squash creates long, spiraling noodles or ribbons. If you find yourself preparing this type of dish many times, it might be a good idea to invest in a vegetable spiralizer. This tool makes perfect thin or thick noodles that can be several feet long, depending on the size and width of your vegetables.

FOR THE DRESSING

1 avocado, peeled, pitted, and chopped

1 tablespoon freshly squeezed lemon juice

1 teaspoon extra-virgin olive oil

2 tablespoons water

2 tablespoons shredded unsweetened coconut

1 tablespoon chopped fresh cilantro

FOR THE NOODLES

4 zucchini, cut into long ribbons with a
    vegetable peeler or spiralizer

Juice of 1 lime

2 cups blanched asparagus, cut into 2-inch pieces

1 cup diced cooked winter squash

TO MAKE THE DRESSING

1. Place the avocado, lemon juice, and olive oil in a blender and blend until smooth.

2. Pour the mixture into a bowl and whisk in the water, coconut, and cilantro until well combined.

3. Set aside. ▸

VEGETARIAN DINNERS

PER SERVING
CALORIES: 188
TOTAL FAT: 14 G
SODIUM: 29 MG
CARBS: 16 G
SUGAR: 6 G
PROTEIN: 5 G

Lime-Coconut Zucchini Noodles with Avocado *continued*

TO MAKE THE NOODLES

1. Toss the zucchini and lime juice in a large bowl until well combined.

2. Let the zucchini stand for 10 minutes.

3. Add the asparagus and squash to the zucchini and toss until well combined.

4. Add the dressing and toss to combine before serving.

VEGETARIAN
DINNERS

"PASTA" WITH SPRING VEGETABLES

KIDS' FAVORITE | QUICK+EASY

▸ Serves 4

▸ Prep time: 20 minutes ▸ Cook time: 10 minutes

The sauce for this "pasta" is a delectable melding of earthy mushrooms, the snap of fresh citrus, and fragrant basil. You might find yourself eating the sauce with a spoon instead of using it for a meal. When you add the green, tender asparagus and swirls of pale zucchini noodles, the dish looks like a picture on the cover of a cooking magazine. The tender stalks of asparagus contain 100 percent of the RDA of vitamin K in just 1 cup. Asparagus is also an excellent source of folate, copper, and vitamins B_1, B_2, and C.

6 zucchini, cut into long ribbons with a vegetable peeler or spiralizer

2 cups asparagus, cut into 3-inch pieces

2 cups halved snap peas

1 tablespoon extra-virgin olive oil

1 cup chopped mushrooms

1 teaspoon minced fresh garlic

1 tablespoon freshly squeezed lemon juice

1 cup shredded spinach

2 tablespoons chopped fresh basil

¼ teaspoon sea salt

VEGETARIAN DINNERS

PER SERVING
CALORIES: 107
TOTAL FAT: 4 G
SODIUM: 184 MG
CARBS: 16 G
SUGAR: 6 G
PROTEIN: 6 G

1. Place a medium pot of water over medium-high heat and bring to a boil.

2. Reduce the heat to medium and blanch the zucchini ribbons for 1 minute. Drain and rinse them immediately under cold water.

3. Pat the ribbons dry with paper towels and transfer the zucchini to a large bowl.

4. Add the asparagus and snap peas to the water and blanch them for 2 minutes.

5. Drain and rinse them immediately under cold water, pat them dry, and add them to the zucchini. Set the bowl aside.

6. Place a large skillet over medium heat and add the olive oil. ▸

"Pasta" with Spring Vegetables *continued*

7. Sauté the mushrooms and garlic until tender, about 3 minutes.

8. Add the lemon juice and spinach and sauté until the spinach is wilted, about 2 minutes.

9. Stir in the basil and salt, then toss the mushroom mixture with the zucchini mixture until they are well combined.

10. Serve immediately.

VEGETARIAN DINNERS

ROASTED SPAGHETTI SQUASH AND KALE

▸ Serves 4

▸ Prep time: 10 minutes ▸ Cook time: 1 hour

Spaghetti squash is a winter squash, and it shreds into spaghetti-like strands when it is cooked. Winter squash should be included regularly as part of a healthy diet because it provides a large amount immune-boosting carotenoids. Winter squash is also an excellent source of vitamins A, B_6, and C as well as fiber and manganese.

1 spaghetti squash (about 5 pounds), halved and seeded

3 teaspoons extra-virgin olive oil

1 cup chopped sweet onion

1 teaspoon minced fresh garlic

4 cups chopped kale

1 tablespoon gluten-free balsamic vinegar

Pinch sea salt

1. Preheat the oven to 350°F.

2. Line a baking sheet with parchment paper.

3. Place the squash, cut-side down, on the baking sheet and lightly brush the skin with 1 teaspoon of olive oil.

4. Bake the squash until it is very tender, about 1 hour.

5. While the squash is baking, place a large skillet on medium-high heat and add the remaining 2 teaspoons of olive oil.

6. Sauté the onion and garlic until the onion is softened, about 3 minutes.

7. Add the kale and sauté until it is wilted, about 5 minutes.

8. Remove the skillet from the heat, stir in the balsamic vinegar, and season with salt. Set aside.

9. When the squash is tender, remove it from the oven and use a fork to scrape out the squash strands from the skin.

10. Put the squash noodles in a large serving bowl and top them with the sautéed kale mixture.

11. Serve immediately.

VEGETARIAN DINNERS

PER SERVING
CALORIES: 257
TOTAL FAT: 7 G
SODIUM: 360 MG
CARBS: 50 G
SUGAR: 2 G
PROTEIN: 6 G

SIMPLE VEGETABLE CURRY

QUICK + EASY

▸ Serves 4

▸ Prep time: 10 minutes ▸ Cook time: 20 minutes

Many of the spices in traditional curry are missing in this dish, but the ones that are used (turmeric, cinnamon, and pungent cloves) create an exotic flavor that is further enhanced by the heat from the fresh ginger. Turmeric adds a peppery, almost citrus accent to curry and is largely responsible for its sunny color. This ancient spice is a powerful anti-inflammatory that may help improve problems related to inflammatory bowel syndrome, rheumatoid arthritis, and cystic fibrosis.

VEGETARIAN
DINNERS

PER SERVING
CALORIES 106
TOTAL FAT: 5 G
SODIUM: 56 MG
CARBS: 15 G
SUGAR: 5 G
PROTEIN: 5 G

1 tablespoon coconut oil

2 cups halved mushrooms

1 sweet onion, sliced thinly

1 teaspoon minced fresh garlic

1 teaspoon grated fresh ginger

4 cups small broccoli florets

1 cup peeled and sliced carrots

1 cup sliced zucchini

½ cup unsweetened organic coconut milk (for homemade, see page 258)

½ teaspoon turmeric

¼ teaspoon ground cinnamon

Pinch ground cloves

2 tablespoons thinly shredded fresh basil

1. Place a large saucepan over medium-high heat and add the coconut oil.

2. Sauté the mushrooms, onion, garlic, and ginger until softened, about 3 minutes.

3. Add the broccoli, carrots, zucchini, coconut milk, turmeric, cinnamon, and cloves, and bring the mixture to a boil.

4. Reduce the heat to low and simmer until the vegetables are tender, about 15 minutes.

5. Stir in the shredded basil and serve immediately.

COCONUT PAD THAI

KIDS' FAVORITE | QUICK+EASY

- ► Serves 4
- ► Prep time: 20 minutes

Made from coconut sap and often used as a soy sauce substitute, coconut aminos can be found in many large grocery store chains and health food stores. It contains an impressive amount of amino acids, vitamin C, and potassium. Coconut aminos may help regulate blood sugar, improve blood pressure, and decrease inflammation in the body. If you like a more intense flavor for your pad thai, you can add 1 teaspoon of fish sauce and omit the sea salt. Be sure to read the label on the fish sauce to ensure it contains no additives that are not allowed on the Autoimmune Paleo Diet.

FOR THE SAUCE

2 tablespoons minced fresh garlic

2 tablespoons maple syrup

1 tablespoon coconut aminos

1 tablespoon chopped fresh cilantro

1 tablespoon extra-virgin olive oil

Dash sea salt

FOR THE VEGETABLES

4 cups shredded Napa cabbage

4 zucchini, cut into long ribbons with a vegetable peeler or spiralizer

3 cups peeled and shredded carrots

½ red onion, very thinly sliced

TO MAKE THE DRESSING

1. Whisk the garlic, maple syrup, coconut aminos, cilantro, and olive oil in a small bowl until well combined.

2. Season the dressing with salt and set aside.

TO MAKE THE VEGETABLES

1. Toss the cabbage, zucchini, carrots, and onion in a large bowl until well combined.

2. Add the dressing and toss to combine before serving.

VEGETARIAN DINNERS

PER SERVING
CALORIES: 134
TOTAL FAT: 4 G
SODIUM: 205 MG
CARBS: 24 G
SUGAR: 14 G
PROTEIN: 4 G

CHAPTER TWELVE

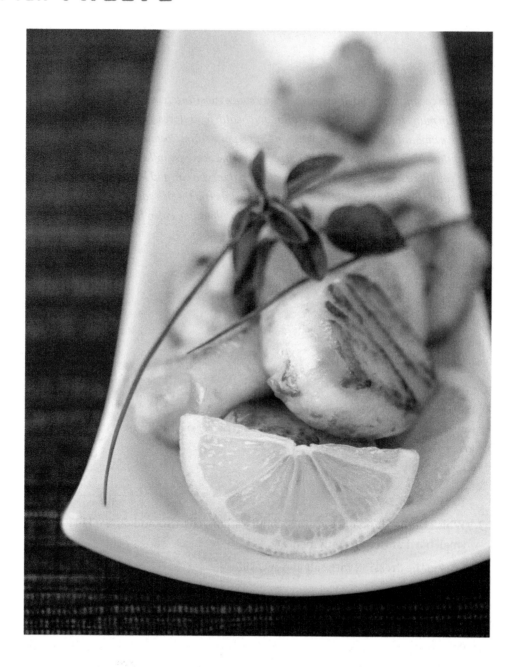

FISH AND SEAFOOD

SHRIMP SCAMPI

▶ Serves 4

▶ Prep time: 15 minutes ▶ Cook time: 10 minutes

Shrimp is very high in selenium, vitamin B_{12}, protein, phosphorus, choline, and copper. This nutrition profile means shrimp may help reduce the risk of cardiovascular disease, type 2 diabetes, and depression. Much of the shrimp available today is farm-raised, but farming techniques have created a poor-quality product. Unfortunately, cultivating shrimp in a more natural open habitat is also creating issues, such as the destruction of ecosystems in the environment. So whenever possible, choose sustainable shrimp that is labeled by an accredited independent agency, such as the Marine Stewardship Council.

FISH AND SEAFOOD

PER SERVING
CALORIES: 127
TOTAL FAT: 4 G
SODIUM: 123 MG
CARBS: 3 G
SUGAR: 0 G
PROTEIN: 22 G

1 tablespoon extra-virgin olive oil

3 teaspoons minced fresh garlic

1 pound (21 to 25 count) shrimp, peeled and deveined

½ cup chopped fresh parsley

Zest of ½ lemon

Juice of 1 lemon

1. Place a large skillet over medium-high heat and add the olive oil.

2. Sauté the garlic until it is fragrant and softened, about 2 minutes.

3. Add the shrimp and sauté until they are just pink and cooked through, about 5 minutes.

4. Remove the skillet from the heat and add the parsley, lemon zest, and lemon juice, and toss to mix.

5. Serve immediately.

SHRIMP PAD THAI

KIDS' FAVORITE

- ▸ Serves 4
- ▸ Prep time: 15 minutes ▸ Cook time: 55 minutes

Pad thai is usually a pan-fried noodle dish with peanuts and lots of heat; it's sweet, sour, spicy, and a little salty. This version is not a traditional pad thai because it uses roasted spaghetti squash instead of noodles and does not contain peanuts, but it does cover the other characteristics of this dish quite well. The honey provides the sweetness, the lime juice is sour, the ginger is mildly hot, and there is a hint of salt in the finished dish.

1 spaghetti squash (about 2 pounds), cut in half and seeded

2 tablespoons coconut oil

½ pound (21 to 25 count) shrimp, peeled and deveined

½ cup chopped sweet onion

2 teaspoons minced fresh garlic

1 teaspoon grated fresh ginger

1 cup peeled and shredded carrots

1 cup julienned green beans

Juice of 1 lime

1 tablespoon local organic honey

1 tablespoon coconut aminos

¼ cup chopped fresh cilantro

FISH AND SEAFOOD

PER SERVING

CALORIES: 222

TOTAL FAT: 8 G

SODIUM: 159 MG

CARBS: 28 G

SUGAR: 7 G

PROTEIN: 15 G

1. Preheat the oven to 400°F.

2. Line a baking sheet with parchment paper.

3. Lightly brush the insides of the squash halves with 1 tablespoon of coconut oil and place them, cut-side down, on the baking sheet.

4. Bake the squash until it is tender, about 45 minutes.

5. Shred the squash into long strands using a fork and transfer the squash to a large bowl. Set aside.

6. Add the remaining 1 tablespoon of coconut oil to a large skillet over medium-high heat. ▸

7. Sauté the shrimp until pink and cooked through, about 5 minutes. Transfer the shrimp to a small bowl and set aside.

8. Add the onion, garlic, and ginger to the skillet and sauté until the onion is softened, about 3 minutes.

9. Add the carrots and green beans and sauté until they are tender-crisp, about 3 minutes.

10. Stir in the spaghetti squash, shrimp, lime juice, honey, coconut aminos, and cilantro.

11. Serve immediately.

FISH AND SEAFOOD

LEMON SCALLOPS

▸ Serves 4

▸ Prep time: 10 minutes ▸ Cook time: 10 minutes

Scallops are one of the easiest and quickest seafood products to cook. Their flavor is sweet and fresh, and this shellfish is available frozen year-round. Scallops are very low in fat and calories and are a rich source of vitamin B$_{12}$, selenium, magnesium, and protein. Eating scallops as part of a healthy diet may reduce the risk of colon cancer and cardiovascular disease.

¼ cup extra-virgin olive oil

2 tablespoons minced fresh garlic

2 pounds cleaned sea scallops

Dash sea salt

2 tablespoons freshly squeezed lemon juice

1 teaspoon lemon zest

1 tablespoon chopped fresh parsley, for garnish

1. Place a large skillet over medium-high heat and add the olive oil.

2. Sauté the garlic until it is fragrant, about 2 minutes.

3. Pat the scallops dry and season them lightly with salt.

4. Add the scallops to the skillet and cook until they are lightly seared and just cooked through, turning once, about 4 minutes per side.

5. Transfer the scallops to a serving plate and set aside.

6. Add the lemon juice and zest to the pan and stir to combine.

7. Spoon the sauce over the scallops.

8. Serve the scallops garnished with fresh parsley.

FISH AND SEAFOOD

PER SERVING

CALORIES: 426

TOTAL FAT: 28 G

SODIUM: 440 MG

CARBS: 7 G

SUGAR: 0 G

PROTEIN: 38 G

TUNA BURGERS

▸ Serves 4

▸ Prep time: 10 minutes, plus 1 hour to chill ▸ Cook time: 10 minutes

Tuna is found on many controversial food lists because of the potential for mercury contamination and the fact it can cause an allergic reaction in some people. The best choices for mercury-free tuna are skipjack and tongol tuna. Always buy your fresh tuna from a reputable fishmonger, and you should not smell a fishy aroma when you bring the tuna fillets up to your nose. All the fish products in the fish counter should be displayed packed in ice or on the ice to preserve freshness.

1 (1-pound) sushi-grade tuna fillet, cut into ¼-inch chunks

2 tablespoons chopped sweet onion

5 teaspoons chopped fresh cilantro

1 tablespoon arrowroot powder

1 teaspoon grated fresh ginger

¼ teaspoon sea salt

1 tablespoon extra-virgin olive oil

1. Mix the tuna, onion, cilantro, arrowroot, ginger, and salt in a medium bowl until well combined.

2. Form the tuna mixture into 4 equal patties, each about ½ inch thick.

3. Place the patties in the refrigerator for 1 hour to firm.

4. Place a large skillet over medium-high heat and add the olive oil.

5. Pan-fry the tuna burgers until they are browned but still slightly pink in the center, turning once, about 8 minutes total.

6. Let the tuna burgers rest for 1 to 2 minutes before serving.

FISH AND SEAFOOD

PER SERVING
CALORIES: 185
TOTAL FAT: 6 G
SODIUM: 118 MG
CARBS: 1 G
SUGAR: 0 G
PROTEIN: 32 G

MAPLE SALMON

- ▶ Serves 4
- ▶ Prep time: 5 minutes ▶ Cook time: 20 minutes

The strong taste of salmon combines well with sweet flavorings such as maple syrup, which creates a gorgeous caramelized crust on the fish. This dish could also be made with honey, but it will not caramelize the same. Try pairing this recipe with a tangy grapefruit salad or simple sautéed vegetables for a light dinner. The best salmon in terms of sustainable fisheries and contamination concerns is wild-caught Alaskan salmon. Wild-caught fish are typically lower in saturated fat, have a healthier omega-6 to omega-3 fatty acids ratio, and are higher in vitamins and minerals than their farmed counterparts.

¼ cup maple syrup

2 tablespoons coconut oil

3 teaspoons freshly squeezed lemon juice

1 teaspoon chopped fresh thyme

4 (6-ounce) salmon fillets

1. Preheat the oven to 400°F.
2. Whisk the maple syrup, coconut oil, lemon juice, and thyme in a small bowl until well combined.
3. Place the salmon fillets on a small baking sheet and pour the glaze over the fish.
4. Bake the salmon until the fish is opaque, about 20 minutes.
5. Serve immediately.

FISH AND SEAFOOD

PER SERVING
CALORIES: 337
TOTAL FAT: 17 G
SODIUM: 78 MG
CARBS: 14 G
SUGAR: 12 G
PROTEIN: 33 G

HERB-CRUSTED SALMON

FODMAP-FREE | QUICK + EASY

▶ Serves 4

▶ Prep time: 10 minutes ▶ Cook time: 20 minutes

Salmon is a forgiving fish to cook in most cases; because it is naturally oily, even when slightly overcooked it is still palatable. If you think you are going to be making a great deal of salmon and are reasonably comfortable with cleaning fish, then buying an entire side or even a whole salmon is more economical than individual fillets. Choose fish with pink, fresh-looking gills, clear eyes, and a smooth, slime-free skin to ensure the salmon is fresh caught.

4 (6-ounce) salmon fillets

1 teaspoon extra-virgin olive oil

2 teaspoons coconut flour

1 tablespoon chopped fresh parsley

1 teaspoon chopped fresh thyme

Pinch sea salt

1. Preheat the oven to 350°F.
2. Line a baking sheet with parchment paper.
3. Place the salmon fillets on the baking sheet and pat them dry with a paper towel.
4. Brush the tops of the salmon with the olive oil.
5. Stir the coconut flour, parsley, thyme, and salt in a small bowl until well combined.
6. Spoon the herb mixture evenly atop the salmon fillets.
7. Bake the salmon until it is opaque, about 20 minutes.
8. Serve immediately.

FISH AND SEAFOOD

PER SERVING

CALORIES: 242

TOTAL FAT: 12 G

SODIUM: 137 MG

CARBS: 1 G

SUGAR: 0 G

PROTEIN: 33 G

SALMON FLORENTINE

QUICK + EASY

- ► Serves 4
- ► Prep time: 5 minutes ► Cook time: 25 minutes

Florentine as a cooking term has come to refer to dishes that contain spinach, like this one. Spinach and other dark leafy greens are often called superfoods. Most greens are an excellent source of vitamins C, E, and K as well as iron, calcium, and potassium. You can replace the spinach here with chard, kale, or a combination of greens.

1 teaspoon coconut oil
2 teaspoons minced fresh garlic
4 cups spinach
4 (6-ounce) salmon fillets
Dash sea salt

1. Preheat the oven to 350°F.
2. Line a baking sheet with parchment paper and set aside.
3. Place a large skillet over medium-high heat and add the coconut oil.
4. Sauté the garlic until softened, about 3 minutes.
5. Add the spinach and sauté until the spinach wilts, about 3 minutes.
6. Remove the skillet from the heat.
7. Place the salmon fillets on the baking sheet and season them with salt.
8. Top the fillets evenly with the spinach mixture.
9. Bake the salmon until it is opaque, about 20 minutes.
10. Serve immediately.

FISH AND SEAFOOD

PER SERVING
CALORIES: 246
TOTAL FAT: 12 G
SODIUM: 158 MG
CARBS: 2 G
SUGAR: 0 G
PROTEIN: 34 G

LIME-INFUSED POACHED SALMON

FODMAP-FREE | MAKE AHEAD | QUICK+EASY

▸ Serves 4

▸ Prep time: 5 minutes ▸ Cook time: 15 minutes

It's convenient to have some poached fish in your refrigerator during the week, because it is so versatile. You can eat it as the main part of the meal or flake it into vegetable dishes, salads, and soups. The salmon fillets will become infused with the flavors of the poaching broth, so try experimenting with different herbs, chopped vegetables, and spices to see which flavors appeal to you.

½ cup water

Juice and zest of 1 lime

2 tablespoons chopped fresh thyme

4 (6-ounce) salmon fillets

FISH AND SEAFOOD

PER SERVING
CALORIES: 229
TOTAL FAT: 11 G
SODIUM: 79 MG
CARBS: 1 G
SUGAR: 0 G
PROTEIN: 33 G

1. Place a large pan that fits all the salmon fillets in one layer over high heat and add the water, juice, zest, and thyme.

2. Add the salmon fillets to the pan and bring the liquid to a boil.

3. Reduce the heat to medium-low and cover the pan, simmering the salmon until it is opaque and cooked through, about 15 minutes.

4. Remove the fillets carefully from the skillet and discard the poaching liquid.

5. Serve the fish hot or cold.

WHOLE GRILLED TROUT WITH HERBS

FODMAP-FREE | QUICK+EASY

- ▸ Serves 4
- ▸ Prep time: 10 minutes ▸ Cook time: 15 minutes

Don't let the thought of fish heads and bones scare you away from trying whole fish. You can choose a fresh trout from your local fishmonger, sometimes right out of a tank filled with swimming fish, and ask for the fish to be completely cleaned for you. This means the scales, head, innards, and even the bones up to the spine are removed. Then all you have to do is stuff, broil, and serve.

1 (2-pound) whole trout, cleaned and scaled

1 tablespoon extra-virgin olive oil

Dash sea salt

½ cup chopped fresh parsley

6 sprigs fresh thyme

2 lemons, 1 sliced and 1 cut into 8 wedges

FISH AND SEAFOOD

PER SERVING
CALORIES: 249
TOTAL FAT: 12 G
SODIUM: 62 MG
CARBS: 1 G
SUGAR: 0 G
PROTEIN: 34 G

1. Preheat the oven to broil.

2. Line a baking sheet with foil. Place a wire rack on the baking sheet.

3. Use a sharp knife to make 6 slashes in the skin on each side of the fish.

4. Rub the fish with olive oil and season both sides lightly with salt.

5. Stuff the cavity of the fish with the parsley, thyme, and lemon slices.

6. Place the fish on the wire rack and broil each side for 8 minutes. Cook the fish a little longer if it does not flake with a fork.

7. Serve the trout with the lemon wedges.

HALIBUT WITH LEEKS

▸ Serves 4

▸ Prep time: 10 minutes ▸ Cook time: 25 minutes

Leeks have a mild, fresh taste that is enhanced when cooked. Leeks are rich in manganese and vitamins B_6 and K. Including leeks as a regular part of your diet may cut your risk of atherosclerosis, type 2 diabetes, and rheumatoid arthritis. Leeks need some extra attention when you are cleaning them, because dirt can be found between all the folds of the stalks. So slice your leeks into thin rounds, dump them into a large bowl or full sink of cold water, and swirl them around, gently rubbing the slices between your fingers. Let the leeks soak for about 5 minutes to allow the heavier dirt to settle before you scoop the floating leeks out of the water.

**FISH AND
SEAFOOD**

PER SERVING
CALORIES: 431
TOTAL FAT: 15G
SODIUM: 686 MG
CARBS: 15 G
SUGAR: 4 G
PROTEIN: 56 G

5 slices organic bacon, diced

½ cup chopped sweet onion

1 teaspoon minced fresh garlic

4 leeks, white and light green parts only, thinly sliced

1 teaspoon chopped fresh thyme

4 (6-ounce) halibut fillets

½ cup Chicken Bone Broth (page 266)

1. Place a large skillet over medium-high heat and sauté the bacon until it is just cooked, about 4 minutes.

2. Add the onion and garlic and sauté until the onion is softened, about 3 minutes.

3. Add the leeks and thyme and sauté until the leeks are tender, about 5 minutes.

4. Transfer the leek mixture to a plate and set aside.

5. Place the halibut fillets in the same skillet and cook for 4 minutes.

6. Turn the fish and add the bacon mixture back to the skillet along the edges of the pan.

7. Add the chicken broth and cook the fish until it flakes easily with a fork, about 5 minutes.

8. Serve the halibut topped with the leek mixture.

COLORFUL CRAB CAKES

MAKE AHEAD | KIDS' FAVORITE | GOOD FOR BATCHES

- ▸ Makes 3 servings
- ▸ Prep time: 20 minutes ▸ Cook time: 12 minutes

Crab cakes look like they should be gracing a plate in an elegant fine dining restaurant, especially when topped with a pretty colorful fruit salsa. Crab is an underused ingredient in most kitchens, which is unfortunate because it is low calorie and packed with nutrients such as omega-3 fatty acids, protein, selenium, and chromium. These crab cakes can be frozen, uncooked, for up to one month and then you can cook them right from frozen for a quick delicious dinner.

12 ounces canned or fresh lump crab, well drained

1 stalk minced celery

½ carrot, minced

½ avocado, mashed

¼ cup minced red onion

2 tablespoons chopped fresh parsley

1 teaspoon minced garlic

½ teaspoon chopped fresh lemon zest

2 tablespoons coconut flour

2 tablespoons unsweetened organic coconut milk

¼ teaspoon sea salt

FISH AND SEAFOOD

PER SERVING
CALORIES: 206
TOTAL FAT: 19G
SODIUM: 823MG
CARBS: 11G
SUGAR: 2G
PROTEIN: 18G

1. In a medium bowl stir together the crab, celery, avocado, onion, parsley, garlic, and lemon zest until the mixture is very well mixed together.

2. Add the coconut flour and stir to combine. Set aside in the fridge for about 30 minutes.

3. Add the coconut milk by teaspoons until the mixture holds together well, then season with salt.

4. Form the crab mixture into 12 medium crab cakes and place them in the fridge for about 30 minutes.

5. Preheat the oven to 400°F and line a baking sheet with foil.

6. Place the crab cakes on the baking sheet and bake in the oven, turning once, until golden, about 10 to 12 minutes.

7. Serve warm.

CHAPTER THIRTEEN

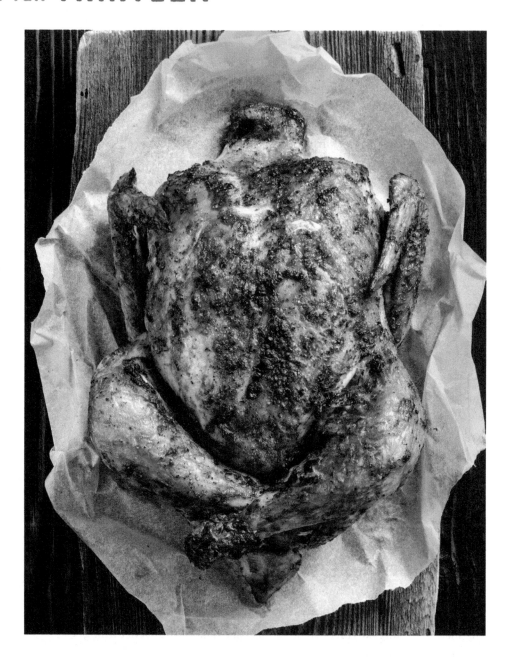

MEAT AND POULTRY

COCONUT CHICKEN CURRY

KIDS' FAVORITE

- ▸ Serves 4
- ▸ Prep time: 15 minutes ▸ Cook time: 45 minutes

This simple stew can be made in a slow cooker, if you want a piping hot meal waiting for you when you get home at the end of the day. Simply combine all the ingredients except the cilantro and salt in a slow cooker and set it on low heat for 8 to 9 hours. Add the remaining ingredients just before you're ready to eat and serve it over Mashed Cauliflower (page 178) for a more substantial meal.

1 tablespoon coconut oil

3 (6-ounce) boneless, skinless chicken breasts, cut into 1-inch chunks

4 teaspoons minced fresh garlic

1 tablespoon grated fresh ginger

1½ cups Chicken Bone Broth (page 266)

1 cup unsweetened organic coconut milk (for homemade, see page 258)

3 celery stalks, chopped

2 cups peeled and diced carrots

1 teaspoon turmeric

3 tablespoons chopped fresh cilantro

¼ teaspoon sea salt

MEAT AND POULTRY

PER SERVING
CALORIES: 326
TOTAL FAT: 14 G
SODIUM: 285 MG
CARBS: 10 G
SUGAR: 3 G
PROTEIN: 38 G

1. Place a large saucepan over medium-high and add the coconut oil.

2. Sauté the chicken until it is lightly browned and almost cooked through, about 5 minutes.

3. Add the garlic and ginger and sauté for 2 minutes.

4. Add the chicken broth, coconut milk, celery, carrots, and turmeric, and bring the curry to a boil, then reduce the heat and simmer, stirring occasionally, until the vegetables and chicken are tender, about 35 minutes.

5. Stir in the cilantro and season with salt.

6. Serve immediately.

SIMPLY PERFECT ROAST CHICKEN

KIDS' FAVORITE | GOOD FOR BATCHES

- ▶ Serves 4
- ▶ Prep time: 10 minutes, plus 15 minutes to stand
- ▶ Cook time: 1 hour, 30 minutes

Roast chicken can be the base of many recipes, from salads to soups and appetizers. To save time, roast two chickens and strip the meat off the unused chicken to save for other meals. Use both chicken carcasses for Chicken Bone Broth (page 266). You can also make this recipe in a slow cooker, but you will end up with chicken that is more stewed than roasted. Slice the onion instead of quartering it and place the onion in the bottom of the slow cooker with the prepared chicken on top. Set your slow cooker on low and cook the chicken for 6 to 8 hours.

1 (4-pound) whole roasting chicken

¾ teaspoon sea salt

1 sweet onion, quartered

3 garlic cloves, lightly smashed

3 sprigs fresh thyme

1 tablespoon extra-virgin olive oil

1. Preheat the oven to 350°F.

2. Wash the chicken in cold water, inside and out, and pat it dry with paper towels.

3. Salt the cavity of the chicken with ½ teaspoon of salt and stuff the cavity with the onion, garlic, and thyme.

4. Place the chicken in a baking dish and brush the skin with the olive oil.

5. Salt the chicken skin with the remaining ¼ teaspoon of salt.

6. Roast the chicken until it is golden brown and cooked through (internal temperature of 185°F), about 1 hour and 30 minutes.

7. Remove the chicken from the oven and let it stand for 15 minutes.

8. Remove the onion, garlic, and thyme, and serve.

MEAT AND POULTRY

PER SERVING
CALORIES: 174
TOTAL FAT: 6 G
SODIUM: 322 MG
CARBS: 3 G
SUGAR: 1 G
PROTEIN: 25 G

ROSEMARY CHICKEN

KIDS' FAVORITE

▸ Serves 4

▸ Prep time: 15 minutes, plus 10 minutes to stand ▸ Cook time: 30 minutes

Fresh rosemary looks like a sprig from an evergreen tree and has a pungent pine-like fragrance when you crush a few needles between your fingers. Rosemary has been used medicinally and in cooking for many centuries. It is thought to stimulate the memory and improve concentration, boost the immune system, and promote healthy digestion. Use fresh rosemary for this dish for a superior taste. Simply wash the entire sprig, strip the needles off the stem, and chop very finely.

2 tablespoons extra-virgin olive oil

Juice of 1 lemon

1 teaspoon minced fresh garlic

1 tablespoon chopped fresh rosemary

4 (8-ounce) boneless, skinless chicken thighs

1. Preheat the oven to 450°F.

2. Whisk 1 tablespoon of olive oil, lemon juice, garlic, and rosemary in a small bowl until well combined. Set aside.

3. Place a large ovenproof skillet over medium-heat and add the remaining 1 tablespoon of olive oil.

4. Sear the chicken thighs for 3 minutes on each side.

5. Add the dressing to the chicken, cover the skillet, and place it in the oven.

6. Roast the chicken until it is cooked through and tender, 20 to 25 minutes.

7. Let the chicken stand for 10 minutes before serving.

MEAT AND POULTRY

PER SERVING
CALORIES: 417
TOTAL FAT: 23 G
SODIUM: 42 MG
CARBS: 1 G
SUGAR: 0 G
PROTEIN: 49 G

LEMON-HERB LAMB CUTLETS

- ▶ Serves 4
- ▶ Prep time: 10 minutes, plus 10 hours to marinate ▶ Cook time: 6 minutes

Lamb cutlets are from the loin of the animal; they are the small bone-in portion that contains the loin and the tenderloin. Ask your butcher to French, or expose the bones, these lean chops for an elegant look. If you like your lamb medium-rare, get these cutlets at least 1 inch thick.

12 lamb cutlets (about 1 pound total)
¼ teaspoon sea salt
½ cup extra-virgin olive oil
¼ cup freshly squeezed lemon juice
2 tablespoons chopped fresh parsley
1 tablespoon chopped fresh thyme

1. Season the lamb chops with salt and place them in 1 layer in a sealable container.

2. Whisk the olive oil, lemon juice, parsley, and thyme in a small bowl until well combined.

3. Pour the marinade over the lamb.

4. Marinate the lamb in the refrigerator for about 10 hours, turning the chops several times.

5. Preheat the barbecue to medium-high.

6. Grill the chops for 2 to 3 minutes per side for medium doneness.

7. If you do not have a barbecue, place a large skillet over medium-high heat and add 1 tablespoon of olive oil. Pan sear the cutlets, in 2 batches if you have to, for about 4 minutes per side for medium doneness.

8. Let the chops rest 5 minutes before serving.

MEAT AND POULTRY

PER SERVING
CALORIES: 277
TOTAL FAT: 16 G
SODIUM: 125 MG
CARBS: 1 G
SUGAR: 0 G
PROTEIN: 32 G

LAMB SLIDERS

MAKE AHEAD | KIDS' FAVORITE | QUICK+EASY | GOOD FOR BATCHES

▸ Serves 4

▸ Prep time: 10 minutes ▸ Cook time: 15 minutes

If you are a beef burger fan, you might find yourself wavering from that devotion when you taste these juicy lamb burgers. It is important to get good-quality, pasture-raised ground lamb from a butcher whenever possible, or grind it yourself, because the ground lamb sold in most supermarkets is high in fat. The herb and spice accents in this recipe are subtle, letting the flavor of the meat take center stage. Cinnamon is a popular spice used to help regulate blood sugar, reduce cholesterol levels, and even help stop some of the damage associated with multiple sclerosis.

MEAT AND POULTRY

PER SERVING
CALORIES: 393
TOTAL FAT: 19 G
SODIUM: 65 MG
CARBS: 4 G
SUGAR: 1 G
PROTEIN: 48 G

4 teaspoons extra-virgin olive oil

1 cup chopped sweet onion

2 teaspoons minced fresh garlic

1½ pounds ground lamb

1 teaspoon grated fresh ginger

½ teaspoon ground cinnamon

½ teaspoon chopped fresh thyme

Dash sea salt

1. Place a small skillet over medium-high heat and add 2 teaspoons of olive oil.

2. Sauté the onions and garlic until tender, about 3 minutes.

3. Transfer the mixture to a medium bowl and let it cool for 10 minutes.

4. Add the lamb, ginger, cinnamon, thyme, and salt to the bowl and mix until well combined.

5. Divide the lamb mixture into 12 equal pieces and form the pieces into ½-inch-thick patties.

6. Place a large skillet over medium-high heat and pan-fry the patties in the remaining 2 teaspoons of olive oil until lightly browned, about 5 minutes per side, for medium-well doneness.

7. Serve immediately.

PEAR-STUFFED PORK LOIN

▸ Serves 6

▸ Prep time: 15 minutes ▸ Cook time: 1 hour

You will be proud to serve slices of this spectacular golden roasted pork loin, featuring spirals of fruit-laced stuffing. Sweet fruit, such as these elegant pears, pairs beautifully with pork. You could also substitute apples or peaches. Pears are high in dietary fiber, vitamins C and K, and copper. This fruit may help protect against cancers such as breast cancer and reduce the risk of degenerative eye diseases.

1 (4-pound) boneless pork loin

1 pear, peeled, cored, and chopped

1 cup chopped mushrooms

¼ cup dried cranberries

¼ cup chopped sweet onion

2 teaspoons minced fresh garlic

1 teaspoon chopped fresh thyme

1 teaspoon chopped fresh parsley

MEAT AND POULTRY

PER SERVING

CALORIES: 454

TOTAL FAT: 11 G

SODIUM: 31 MG

CARBS: 5 G

SUGAR: 3 G

PROTEIN: 80 G

1. Preheat the oven to 325°F.

2. Cut the pork loin lengthwise through the middle, leaving 2 inches connected all the way down the length. Open the loin up like a book, then cut each side horizontally almost all the way through so that you can unfold the pork almost flat. Set aside.

3. Stir the pear, mushrooms, cranberries, onion, garlic, thyme, and parsley in a medium bowl until well combined.

4. Spread the pear mixture evenly over the pork and roll the pork up tightly.

5. Tie the pork roll with kitchen twine at 2-inch intervals to hold it together.

6. Place the tied loin on a baking tray and roast it until the loin is cooked through (internal temperature of 145°F), about 1 hour.

7. Remove the string and serve.

PORK CHOPS WITH MUSHROOMS

KIDS' FAVORITE

▸ Serves 4

▸ Prep time: 10 minutes ▸ Cook time: 25 minutes

Pork once had a reputation for being a somewhat less healthy choice than chicken; however, it is comparable to chicken in its nutrition, with about the same calories and 1 gram of saturated fat per 3-ounce portion. Pork has less cholesterol than chicken and is a better source of protein. As with all meat choices on the Autoimmune Paleo Diet, it is important to buy organic pork when possible.

4 (5-ounce) bone-in center-cut pork chops

¼ teaspoon sea salt

1 tablespoon extra-virgin olive oil

1 cup chopped sweet onion

1 tablespoon minced fresh garlic

16 ounces sliced mixed mushrooms

1 teaspoon chopped fresh thyme or ½ teaspoon dried thyme

½ cup Chicken Bone Broth (page 266)

1. Pat the pork chops dry with paper towels and season them with salt.

2. Place a large skillet over medium-high heat and add the olive oil.

3. Sear the pork chops on both sides, about 3 minutes per side.

4. Transfer the chops to a plate.

5. Add the onion and garlic to the skillet and sauté for 3 minutes.

6. Add the mushrooms and thyme and sauté until the mushrooms are tender, about 5 minutes.

7. Add the chicken broth and pork chops, cover the skillet, reduce the heat, and simmer until the pork is cooked through, about 10 minutes.

8. Serve the pork chops with the sauce spooned on top.

MEAT AND POULTRY

PER SERVING
CALORIES: 311
TOTAL FAT: 16 G
SODIUM: 140 MG
CARBS: 8 G
SUGAR: 3 G
PROTEIN: 33 G

GRILLED HERBED PORK TENDERLOIN

QUICK+EASY

▶ Serves 4

▶ Prep time: 10 minutes, plus 4 hours to marinate ▶ Cook time: 20 minutes

Oregano is an excellent source of vitamin K and fiber and is a powerful antibacterial and antioxidant. If you want an even more delicious marinade for your pork tenderloin, try roasting the garlic before adding it to the other marinade ingredients. Cut the top ½ inch off a head of garlic to expose the cloves and drizzle the head with extra-virgin olive oil. Place the garlic head on a baking sheet and roast it in a 350°F oven until it's very tender and fragrant, about 30 minutes. Squeeze out about six cloves for this marinade and save the rest for another recipe.

4 garlic cloves, peeled

¼ cup chopped fresh oregano or 2 tablespoons dried oregano

¼ cup freshly squeezed orange juice

2 tablespoons lemon zest

2 tablespoons extra-virgin olive oil

1 pound pork tenderloin

MEAT AND POULTRY

PER SERVING
CALORIES: 263
TOTAL FAT: 11 G
SODIUM: 66 MG
CARBS: 9 G
SUGAR: 2 G
PROTEIN: 30 G

1. Place the garlic, oregano, orange juice, lemon zest, and olive oil in a blender and pulse until the marinade is smooth.

2. Pour the marinade in a sealable plastic bag and add the pork tenderloin.

3. Seal the bag, after removing as much air as possible, and marinate the pork in the refrigerator, turning the bag a few times, for 4 hours.

4. Preheat the barbecue to medium-high heat.

5. Remove the tenderloin from the marinade and discard the marinade.

6. Grill the pork, turning several times, until it is just slightly pink (internal temperature of 160°F), about 20 minutes.

7. If you do not have a barbecue, preheat the oven to 400°F and place an oven-safe skillet over medium-high heat on your stove top. Sear the pork tenderloin on all sides, about 3 minutes total, then place the whole skillet in the oven and roast the pork until just cooked through, about 25 minutes.

8. Let the meat stand for 10 minutes before serving.

FLANK STEAK WITH LIME MARINADE

- ▶ Serves 4
- ▶ Prep time: 5 minutes, plus 2 hours to marinate ▶ Cook time: 10 minutes

Flank steak is not an expensive cut of beef, so it is usually marinated and sliced very thinly before serving. This cut comes from the abdominal area of the animal and is characterized by long visible muscle fibers. The lime and garlic marinade infuses a Southwestern flavor to the meat that works well paired with Minted Radish Salad (page 171).

Juice of 2 limes

4 tablespoons freshly squeezed orange juice

2 teaspoons apple cider vinegar

2 teaspoons minced fresh garlic

1 teaspoon grated fresh ginger

1½ pounds flank steak

1. Whisk the lime juice, orange juice, vinegar, garlic, and ginger in a small bowl until well combined.

2. Pour the marinade into a sealable plastic bag and add the steak.

3. Seal the bag, after removing as much air as possible, and marinate the steak in the refrigerator for at least 2 hours.

4. Preheat the barbecue to medium-high heat.

5. Remove the steak from the marinade and discard the marinade.

6. Grill the steak for 5 minutes per side for medium doneness.

7. If you do not have a barbecue, preheat the oven to broil and broil the steak until it is the desired doneness, about 5 minutes per side for medium doneness.

8. Let the steak stand for 10 minutes before slicing it thinly across the grain and serving.

MEAT AND POULTRY

PER SERVING

CALORIES: 341

TOTAL FAT: 14 G

SODIUM: 96 MG

CARBS: 2 G

SUGAR: 1 G

PROTEIN: 48 G

SALISBURY STEAK

KIDS' FAVORITE

▶ Serves 4

▶ Prep time: 15 minutes ▶ Cook time: 30 minutes

Salisbury steak is just a fancy way to describe beef patties covered with sauce or gravy. This name came from the surname of the American doctor who developed this dish for a low-carbohydrate diet in the 1890s. The lightly caramelized mushrooms in the sauce are not traditional, but they add rich flavor and texture.

2 tablespoons extra-virgin olive oil

¼ cup chopped sweet onion

1 teaspoon minced fresh garlic

1½ pounds lean ground beef

Dash sea salt

1 cup sliced button mushrooms

2 cups Easy Beef Bone Broth (page 268)

¼ cup water

1 tablespoon arrowroot powder

MEAT AND POULTRY

PER SERVING
CALORIES: 395
TOTAL FAT: 18 G
SODIUM: 87 MG
CARBS: 4 G
SUGAR: 1 G
PROTEIN: 52 G

1. Place a large skillet over medium-high heat and add 1 tablespoon of olive oil.

2. Sauté the onion and garlic until softened, about 3 minutes.

3. Remove the skillet from the heat and transfer the vegetables to a medium bowl.

4. Add the ground beef and salt to the bowl and mix until well combined.

5. Divide the beef mixture into 4 equal-size patties, each ¾ inch thick.

6. Place the skillet back on the heat and add the remaining 1 tablespoon of olive oil.

7. Sauté the mushrooms until tender and golden, about 5 minutes. Transfer the mushrooms to a plate.

8. Brown the beef patties in the skillet, about 4 minutes per side. ▶

9. Add the beef broth, bring the liquid to a boil, reduce the heat, and simmer, covered, until the patties are cooked through, about 10 minutes.

10. Transfer the patties to a serving plate and cover the plate loosely with foil to keep warm.

11. Whisk the water and arrowroot until smooth and add the arrowroot paste to the broth left in the pan. Whisk the mixture until the sauce is thickened, about 1 minute.

12. Add the mushrooms to the sauce and stir to combine.

13. Pour the sauce over the patties and serve.

MEAT AND POULTRY

SIMPLE BEEF BRISKET

KIDS' FAVORITE

▶ Serves 6

▶ Prep time: 15 minutes ▶ Cook time: 5 hours, 15 minutes

The trick to making a fork-tender brisket is to cook this cut of beef very slowly and for a long time. If you rush the process, the beef will end up tough, so allot enough time for the meat to cook. Make sure you leave the fat cap on the brisket when you cook it, because it helps keep the meat moist.

1 tablespoon extra-virgin olive oil

1 (1½-pound) beef brisket

½ teaspoon sea salt

2 cups thinly sliced sweet onions

4 cups Easy Beef Bone Broth (page 268)

4 teaspoons minced fresh garlic

4 carrots, peeled and cut into 1-inch chunks

3 parsnips, peeled and cut into 1-inch chunks

MEAT AND POULTRY

PER SERVING

CALORIES: 394

TOTAL FAT: 17 G

SODIUM: 167 MG

CARBS: 23 G

SUGAR: 7 G

PROTEIN: 35 G

1. Place a large stockpot over medium-high heat and add the olive oil.

2. Season the brisket with salt and place it in the stockpot.

3. Brown all the sides of the brisket, about 12 minutes total.

4. Remove the stockpot from the heat and transfer the brisket to a plate.

5. Spread the onions in the bottom of the stockpot and place the roast on the onions, fat-side up.

6. Add the beef broth, garlic, carrots, and parsnips to the stockpot.

7. Place the stockpot over medium-high heat and bring the liquid to a boil, then reduce the heat to low, cover, and simmer until the beef is very tender, about 5 hours.

8. Serve the brisket with the vegetables and broth from the pot.

TRADITIONAL BEEF HAMBURGERS

MAKE AHEAD | *KIDS' FAVORITE* | *QUICK+EASY* | GOOD FOR BATCHES

▶ Serves 4

▶ Prep time: 10 minutes ▶ Cook time: 10 minutes

Burgers have a bad reputation with professional nutritionists due to low-quality fast-food offerings and the fact that many burgers are topped with fatty toppings and placed between nutrition-deficient white bread buns. These burgers are all about quality beef accented with a perfect balance of seasonings and topped simply with fresh vegetables.

1½ pounds lean ground beef

½ cup chopped sweet onions

1 teaspoon minced fresh garlic

½ teaspoon chopped fresh thyme

Dash sea salt

4 lettuce leaves

½ red onion, sliced into ¼-inch rounds

1. Mix the ground beef, onions, garlic, thyme, and salt in medium bowl until well combined.

2. Divide the meat mixture into 4 equal pieces and form the pieces into ½-inch-thick patties.

3. Preheat the barbecue to medium-high heat.

4. Grill the burgers until cooked through and lightly charred, turning once, about 5 minutes per side.

5. If you do not have a barbecue, place a large skillet over medium-high heat and add 1 tablespoon of olive oil. Pan sear the burgers until they are cooked through, about 6 minutes per side.

6. Remove the burgers from the grill or skillet and serve them on the lettuce leaves topped with red onion slices.

MEAT AND POULTRY

PER SERVING

CALORIES: 330

TOTAL FAT: 11 G

SODIUM: 87 MG

CARBS: 3 G

SUGAR: 1 G

PROTEIN: 52 G

BEEF STROGANOFF

MAKE AHEAD | GOOD FOR BATCHES

▸ Serves 4

▸ Prep time: 15 minutes ▸ Cook time: 20 minutes

This version of beef stroganoff has an intense beef flavor, but the sauce is more of a broth. Grass-fed beef is the preferred animal choice on the Autoimmune Paleo Diet; it's best because grass-fed beef is lower in cholesterol and higher in beta-carotene and lutein than commercially raised animals. If you want a creamier stroganoff, you can replace the coconut milk in this recipe with ½ cup more bone broth and stir in ½ cup of thick dairy-free coconut yogurt just before serving to mimic the traditional sour cream. Either variation is delicious, but the thicker sauce would be lovely if you serve the stew over Mashed Cauliflower (page 178) or zucchini noodles.

2 tablespoons extra-virgin olive oil

1 pound top sirloin steak, cut into thin strips

1 cup sliced button mushrooms

1 sweet onion, chopped

2 teaspoons minced fresh garlic

1 cup Easy Beef Bone Broth (page 268)

1 cup unsweetened organic coconut milk (for homemade, see page 258)

2 tablespoons chopped fresh parsley, for garnish

1. Place a large skillet over medium-high heat and add the olive oil.

2. Sauté the steak strips until they are lightly browned, about 2 minutes.

3. Transfer the beef to a plate and set aside.

4. Add the mushrooms to the skillet and sauté until tender, about 5 minutes.

5. Transfer the mushrooms to the same plate as the beef.

6. Add the onion and garlic to the skillet and sauté until softened, about 3 minutes.

7. Add the beef broth, coconut milk, beef, mushrooms, and any accumulated juices to the skillet and simmer the stroganoff until the beef is tender, about 10 minutes.

8. Serve the stroganoff garnished with parsley.

MEAT AND POULTRY

PER SERVING

CALORIES: 305

TOTAL FAT: 1 G

SODIUM: 41 MG

CARBS: 5 G

SUGAR: 2 G

PROTEIN: 35 G

POT ROAST

▸ Serves 6

▸ Prep time: 10 minutes ▸ Cook time: 8 hours

There is no need to give up traditional family favorites when you are following the Autoimmune Paleo Diet. Pot roast is a Sunday dinner staple in many households, and this recipe delivers tender slices of meat, beef broth–infused vegetables, and a complex herbed gravy. Simply prepare the casserole dish in the morning and pop it in the oven before going to work. It will be ready to eat after slow roasting in the oven all day.

MEAT AND POULTRY

PER SERVING
CALORIES: 352
TOTAL FAT: 13 G
SODIUM: 120 MG
CARBS: 6 G
SUGAR: 2 G
PROTEIN: 51 G

3 carrots, peeled and cut into 1-inch chunks

2 celery stalks, cut into 2-inch pieces

1 sweet onion, cut into 8 wedges

4 garlic cloves, slightly smashed

2 sprigs fresh thyme

⅓ cup Easy Beef Bone Broth (page 268)

1 (2-pound) chuck roast

¼ teaspoon sea salt

1. Preheat the oven to 275°F.

2. Place the carrots, celery, onion, garlic, thyme, and broth in a large casserole dish.

3. Season the roast with sea salt and place the roast on top of the vegetables.

4. Cover the casserole dish with a lid and roast it until the meat can be shredded with a fork, about 8 hours.

5. Remove the meat and vegetables from the casserole to a serving plate and discard the herb sprigs.

6. Pour the juices from the casserole over the roast before serving.

BACON-WRAPPED VENISON

FODMAP-FREE | QUICK+EASY

- ▸ Serves 4
- ▸ Prep time: 10 minutes ▸ Cook time: 15 minutes

Venison is a very lean meat that benefits from the added fat from the bacon wrapping. Venison is a popular choice for people who are trying to eat only pasture-raised animals, because in most cases, even farm-raised deer are allowed to roam freely. Venison is a complete protein because it contains all the essential amino acids.

4 (5-ounce) venison steaks

¼ teaspoon sea salt

8 slices organic bacon

2 tablespoons extra-virgin olive oil

MEAT AND POULTRY

PER SERVING

CALORIES: 477

TOTAL FAT: 26 G

SODIUM: 167 MG

CARBS: 1 G

SUGAR: 0 G

PROTEIN: 56 G

1. Preheat the oven to 450°F.
2. Season the venison steaks with salt.
3. Wrap each steak around the edges with 2 slices of bacon and secure the bacon with toothpicks.
4. Place a large skillet over medium-high heat and add the olive oil.
5. Place the steaks in the skillet and sear each side for 4 minutes.
6. Transfer the steaks to a baking tray and roast the venison for 6 minutes for medium doneness.
7. Remove the steaks from the oven and let the meat rest for 10 minutes.
8. Remove the toothpicks and serve.

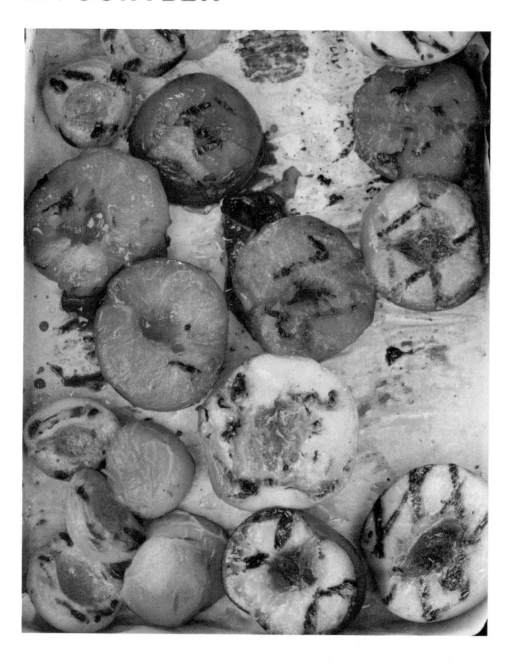

DESSERTS

TROPICAL FRUIT ICE POPS

MAKE AHEAD | KIDS' FAVORITE | QUICK+EASY

- ▸ Makes 8 ice pops
- ▸ Prep time: 10 minutes, plus 3 to 4 hours to chill

Ice pops might not seem like a very elegant dessert, but the exotic fruit in these sunny treats elevates them. You can even add a little coconut milk to enhance the tropical theme. If you can't find a good-quality ripe pineapple, canned fruit packed in juice in a BPA-free can will do. Pineapples do not continue to ripen after they are picked, so take the time to smell the fruit close to the leaves to determine if it is ripe. If the pineapple has a sweet, fragrant scent, it is ready to be eaten.

1 mango, peeled, pitted, and cut into chunks
1 papaya, peeled, seeded, and cut into chunks
½ cup diced fresh pineapple
½ cup water
Juice of 1 lime

1. Place the mango, papaya, pineapple, water, and lime juice in a food processor or blender and process until smooth.

2. Divide the mixture equally among 8 ice pop molds.

3. Freeze the ice pops for 3 to 4 hours before serving.

4. Store the ice pops in the freezer for up to 1 week.

DESSERTS

PER SERVING
CALORIES: 50
TOTAL FAT: 1 G
SODIUM: 4 MG
CARBS: 10 G
SUGAR: 8 G
PROTEIN: 0 G

STRAWBERRY SORBET

▸ Serves 4

▸ Prep time: 10 minutes, plus 1 hour to chill

You don't need an ice cream maker to make this creamy cold dessert. The chunks of fresh strawberries add an interesting texture to this dish and double the berry flavor. This recipe would be nice with an assortment of berries, so experiment with blueberries, blackberries, and raspberries to get delicious variations.

2 cups frozen strawberries

½ avocado, peeled and pitted

¼ cup unsweetened organic coconut milk (for homemade, see page 258)

½ cup chopped fresh strawberries

1. Place the frozen strawberries and avocado in a blender and blend until thick and creamy, about 4 minutes.

2. Add the coconut milk and pulse until well combined.

3. Transfer the mixture to a bowl and stir in the fresh strawberries.

4. Place the sorbet in the freezer in a sealed container for 1 hour before serving.

5. Store leftover sorbet in a sealed container in the freezer for up to 1 month.

DESSERTS

PER SERVING

CALORIES: 85

TOTAL FAT: 5 G

SODIUM: 3 MG

CARBS: 10 G

SUGAR: 5 G

PROTEIN: 1 G

WATERMELON GRANITA

MAKE AHEAD | KIDS' FAVORITE | QUICK+EASY | GOOD FOR BATCHES

▸ Serves 4

▸ Prep time: 15 minutes, plus 8 hours to freeze ▸ Cook time: 15 minutes

Granita is an adult version of a snow cone, but it's an enchanting dessert to serve for children, too. This recipe is also delicious with cantaloupe or honeydew, or a mixture of several types of melons. Use seedless watermelon or you will have to pass the puréed melon through a fine sieve to catch the chopped-up seeds.

1 cup water

6 fresh mint leaves

4 cups cubed watermelon

1 English cucumber, peeled and diced

Juice of 1 lemon

1. Place the water and mint in a saucepan over medium-high heat and bring to a boil. Reduce the heat to low and simmer for 15 minutes to infuse the water with the mint.

2. Strain out the mint leaves and chill the water in the refrigerator for 10 minutes.

3. Add the watermelon and cucumber to a food processor or blender and process until smooth.

4. Add the mint-infused water and lemon juice to the puréed melon mixture and stir until well combined.

5. Pour the melon mixture into a 9-by-13-inch metal baking dish.

6. Place the dish in the freezer for 2 hours.

7. Stir the mixture, scraping the sides, then return the container to the freezer.

8. Scrape the sides and bottom with a spoon every hour until it starts to freeze solid, about 8 hours.

9. When the mixture is almost completely frozen, use a fork to scrape until the watermelon mixture resembles flavored snow before serving.

10. Store the granita in a sealed container in the freezer for up to 1 month.

DESSERTS

PER SERVING

CALORIES: 54

TOTAL FAT: 0 G

SODIUM: 8 MG

CARBS: 14 G

SUGAR: 9 G

PROTEIN: 2 G

FRUIT SALAD WITH LIME

MAKE AHEAD | KIDS' FAVORITE | QUICK+EASY

▸ Serves 4
▸ Prep time: 15 minutes, plus 1 hour to chill

Fruit does not need any enhancements to be exceptional. This glorious salad could be served at the end of a casual summer get-together and would also not be out of place spooned into delicate dishes after a sumptuous fine-dining experience. If you need a slightly more elegant look, try using a melon baller for the watermelon.

2 cups cubed watermelon

2 plums, halved, pitted, and cut into eighths

1 cup halved strawberries

1 cup blackberries

1 cup blueberries

1 tablespoon chopped fresh mint

1 teaspoon lime zest

1. Toss the watermelon, plums, strawberries, blackberries, blueberries, mint, and lime zest in a large bowl.

2. Chill the salad in the refrigerator for 1 hour before serving.

DESSERTS

PER SERVING
CALORIES 78
TOTAL FAT: 0 G
SODIUM: 2 MG
CARBS: 19 G
SUGAR: 13 G
PROTEIN: 2 G

CINNAMON-INFUSED ORANGES AND KIWIS

FODMAP-FREE | MAKE AHEAD | QUICK + EASY

▸ Serves 4
▸ Prep time: 10 minutes, plus 1 hour to marinate

The humble orange becomes something truly special when subtly infused with cinnamon. Oranges are one of the most popular fruits in the world. They are in season and especially sweet in the winter, which is wonderful when you want a bit of fresh sweetness in the gloomy cold months.

2 teaspoons freshly squeezed lemon juice
½ teaspoon ground cinnamon
2 navel oranges, peeled
3 kiwis, peeled and diced

1. Whisk the lemon juice and cinnamon in a medium bowl until well combined and set aside.

2. Cut the oranges into ¼-inch slices.

3. Place the oranges and kiwis in the bowl with the juice mixture and toss to combine.

4. Place the bowl in the refrigerator for at least 1 hour to infuse the flavors before serving.

5. Store the oranges and kiwis in a sealed container in the refrigerator for up to 2 days.

DESSERTS

PER SERVING
CALORIES 79
TOTAL FAT: 0 G
SODIUM: 2 MG
CARBS: 19 G
SUGAR: 14 G
PROTEIN: 2 G

HONEYED CARROT MOUSSE

MAKE AHEAD | *KIDS' FAVORITE* | *QUICK+EASY*

▸ Serves 4

▸ Prep time: 10 minutes, plus 1 hour to chill

Carrot is sweet enough to be served as a dessert and is often found in cakes, puddings, and cookies. If you want your mousse to be sublimely smooth, cook your carrots well so that there is no crunch. You can also pass the puréed mixture through a medium-fine sieve to catch any bits.

2 cups mashed cooked carrots

1 avocado, peeled, pitted, and cut into quarters

¼ cup unsweetened organic coconut milk (for homemade, see page 258)

2 tablespoons unflavored gelatin

1 tablespoon local organic honey

1 teaspoon ground cinnamon

1. Place the carrot, avocado, coconut milk, gelatin, honey, and cinnamon in a food processor or a blender and process until silky smooth.

2. Spoon the mousse into a 6-cup serving bowl and place it in the refrigerator for 1 hour to set before serving.

3. Store the mousse in a sealed container in the refrigerator for up to 2 days.

DESSERTS

PER SERVING

CALORIES: 157

TOTAL FAT: 10 G

SODIUM: 49 MG

CARBS: 15 G

SUGAR: 7 G

PROTEIN: 4 G

BANANA-CAROB PUDDING

FODMAP-FREE | MAKE AHEAD | KIDS' FAVORITE

► Serves 4

► Prep time: 15 minutes, plus 8 hours to chill ► Cook time: 5 minutes

The edible pod of a shrub in the pea family, carob's main benefit to the Auto-immune Paleo Diet is that it tastes a bit like chocolate without the addition of the caffeine and theobromine found in chocolate. Carob is high in fiber, calcium, potassium, and phosphorous. Bananas are available year-round, and you can freeze your ripe bananas in their skin to ensure you always have some on hand for this delectable dessert. Bananas provide potassium, vitamin B_6, and fiber, which means they support a healthy cardiovascular system and may reduce the risk of digestive issues.

DESSERTS

PER SERVING
CALORIES: 144
TOTAL FAT: 6 G
SODIUM: 26 MG
CARBS: 20 G
SUGAR: 11 G
PROTEIN: 3 G

1½ cups unsweetened organic coconut milk (for homemade, see page 258)
1 tablespoon unflavored gelatin
2 very ripe bananas
¼ cup carob powder

1. Stir ½ cup of coconut milk and the gelatin in a small bowl until well combined. Let the mixture sit for 10 minutes.

2. Pour the remaining 1 cup of coconut milk in a saucepan set over medium heat, and cook until it is just heated but not boiling, about 3 minutes.

3. Whisk the gelatin mixture into the hot coconut milk.

4. Place the bananas, carob powder, and hot coconut milk mixture in a blender and process for 30 seconds.

5. Transfer the pudding mixture to a large serving bowl or 4 individual serving bowls.

6. Chill the pudding in the refrigerator for at least 8 hours to set before serving.

7. Store the pudding in a sealed container in the refrigerator for up to 2 days.

SPICE COOKIES

MAKE AHEAD | KIDS' FAVORITE | QUICK+EASY | GOOD FOR BATCHES

- ▶ Makes 12 cookies (2 cookies per serving)
- ▶ Prep time: 10 minutes ▶ Cook time: 20 minutes

Your grandmother's cookies might have tasted similar to these. The classic combination of the spices paired with chewy coconut and sweet dates creates a simple dessert you can stick in your pocket and take with you. This recipe can be doubled (or tripled) easily, and you can freeze the extra cookies in a sealed container for up to 3 months.

¾ cup dates
¼ cup boiling water
⅓ cup puréed pumpkin
1 cup shredded unsweetened coconut
¾ teaspoon ground cinnamon
¼ teaspoon ground ginger
Pinch ground cloves
Pinch sea salt

1. Preheat the oven to 325°F. Line a baking sheet with parchment paper and set aside.

2. Place the dates and boiling water in a small bowl and let stand for 15 minutes.

3. Place the pumpkin, dates (with water), coconut, cinnamon, ginger, cloves, and salt in a food processor or blender and pulse until well combined, about 2 minutes.

4. Use a tablespoon to drop the cookie-size portions of the mixture onto the baking sheet.

5. Flatten the cookies out to ½ inch thick.

6. Bake the cookies until they are firm, about 20 minutes.

7. Let the cookies cool for 10 minutes, then remove them from the baking sheet.

8. Let the cookies cool completely before storing them in a sealed container in the refrigerator for up to 5 days.

DESSERTS

PER SERVING
CALORIES: 101
TOTAL FAT: 6 G
SODIUM: 24 MG
CARBS: 12 G
SUGAR: 8 G
PROTEIN: 1 G

COCONUT SNOWBALLS

MAKE AHEAD | *KIDS' FAVORITE* | *QUICK+EASY* | GOOD FOR BATCHES

- ▸ Makes 12 balls (1 cookie per serving)
- ▸ Prep time: 15 minutes, plus 45 minutes to chill ▸ Cook time: 5 minutes

These charming, frilly cookies can be the perfect accompaniment to a nice cup of herbal tea at the end of a good meal. The warm flavor of cinnamon is familiar to most people, and it is packed with nutritional benefits. Cinnamon is high in manganese and is a good source of fiber and calcium.

1½ cups shredded unsweetened coconut
1 cup Coconut Butter (page 257)
¼ cup local organic honey
¼ teaspoon ground cinnamon

1. Preheat the oven to 350°F.
2. Spread out ½ cup of shredded coconut on a baking sheet.
3. Lightly brown the coconut in the oven, about 5 minutes. Set aside.
4. Mix the coconut butter, the remaining 1 cup of shredded coconut, honey, and cinnamon in a medium bowl until well combined.
5. Chill the mixture for about 45 minutes until it can be rolled into balls.
6. Roll the mixture into 12 balls, then roll the balls in the toasted coconut.
7. Store the coconut balls in a sealed container in the refrigerator for up to 1 week.

DESERTS

PER SERVING
CALORIES: 181
TOTAL FAT: 15 G
SODIUM: 9 MG
CARBS: 12 G
SUGAR: 8 G
PROTEIN: 2 G

APPLE CRUMBLE

MAKE AHEAD | KIDS' FAVORITE

▸ Serves 6

▸ Prep time: 20 minutes ▸ Cook time: 20 minutes

Many traditional crumble recipes are more about the crumble topping than the fruit layer underneath. This healthy crumble is mostly apple with only a scant layer of crunchy topping for texture and a hint of sweetness. Pears, or a combination of pears and apples, would also be a tempting choice for this warm, comforting dessert.

FOR THE FILLING

1½ pounds apples (about 4 large), peeled, cored, and cut into ¼-inch slices

1 teaspoon ground cinnamon

½ teaspoon ground cloves

Pinch sea salt

Pinch ground ginger

FOR THE TOPPING

½ cup coconut flour

¾ cup shredded unsweetened coconut

3 tablespoons Coconut Butter (page 257)

1 tablespoon maple syrup

1 teaspoon ground cinnamon

DESSERTS

PER SERVING

CALORIES: 235

TOTAL FAT: 8 G

SODIUM: 66 MG

CARBS: 39 G

SUGAR: 17 G

PROTEIN: 2 G

TO MAKE THE FILLING

1. Preheat the oven to 350°F.

2. Lightly grease a 9-by-13-inch baking dish with coconut oil and set aside.

3. Mix the apples, cinnamon, cloves, salt, and ginger in a medium bowl until well combined.

4. Transfer the apple mixture to the baking dish and spread it out evenly. ▸

Apple Crumble *continued*

TO MAKE THE TOPPING

1. Mix the coconut flour, coconut, coconut butter, maple syrup, and cinnamon in a bowl until well combined and the mixture resembles crumbs.

2. Sprinkle the topping on the apples.

3. Bake the apples until they are tender and the topping is golden brown, about 20 minutes.

4. Serve the apples warm.

DESSERTS

SPICED APPLESAUCE

▶ Serves 6

▶ Prep time: 10 minutes ▶ Cook time: 20 minutes

The best apples for this dish are tart, crisp varieties such as McIntosh or Cortland, because the finished product tastes more complex with just a hint of tartness. Apples are a low-calorie, nutrient-dense fruit that contains almost every vitamin and mineral in some quantity. Apples are wonderful detoxifiers and are packed with healthy fiber.

2 pounds apples (6 medium), peeled, cored, and chopped

½ cup water

1 teaspoon ground cinnamon

1. Place the apples, water, and cinnamon in a medium saucepan over medium heat and cook until the apples are very tender, stirring occasionally, about 20 minutes.

2. Remove the saucepan from the heat and mash the apples with a potato masher until the applesauce is the desired consistency.

3. Eat the applesauce warm or chilled.

4. Store the applesauce in a sealed container in the refrigerator for up to 1 week.

DESSERTS

PER SERVING

CALORIES: 80

TOTAL FAT: 0 G

SODIUM: 2 MG

CARBS: 21 G

SUGAR: 15 G

PROTEIN: 0 G

GRILLED PEACHES AND APRICOTS

- ▶ Serves 4
- ▶ Prep time: 10 minutes ▶ Cook time: 5 minutes

The flavor of stone fruits is intensified when they are lightly grilled, bringing all the sweetness to the forefront. Peaches in particular get almost candy-like when cooked, if they are perfectly ripe. Plums would be a nice addition to this dish if you want more variety. Picking a perfect peach is as simple as lifting the fruit to your nose and inhaling. Ripe peaches have a heady fragrance that permeates the skin, so if you can't smell anything, put the peach back in the pile. Also, ripe peaches should give slightly when you gently press the skin with your fingertips.

DESSERTS

2 peaches, halved and pitted

4 apricots, halved and pitted

1 tablespoon melted coconut oil

1 teaspoon ground cinnamon

PER SERVING
CALORIES 67
TOTAL FAT: 4 G
SODIUM: 0 MG
CARBS: 9 G
SUGAR: 7 G
PROTEIN: 1 G

1. Preheat the barbecue to medium.

2. Brush the cut edges of the peaches and apricots with the coconut oil.

3. Sprinkle the peaches and apricots with cinnamon.

4. Grill the fruit, cut-side down, until they are lightly charred and tender, about 5 minutes.

5. If you do not have a barbecue, preheat the oven to broil and broil the fruit, cut-side up, until they are tender and lightly browned, about 5 minutes.

6. Serve the peaches and apricots warm.

BAKED CINNAMON BANANAS

▸ Serves 4

▸ Prep time: 10 minutes ▸ Cook time: 20 minutes

Bananas have an almost creamy pudding-like consistency when baked, which contrasts nicely with the crackly sweet crust the honey forms in this recipe. You can make this dish ahead of time and store it, covered, in the refrigerator for up to 2 days before baking it. This sweet treat would also make a lovely breakfast side dish, paired with Simple Pork Sausage (page 127) or a couple strips of organic bacon.

2 tablespoons melted coconut oil

2 tablespoons freshly squeezed lemon juice

1 teaspoon local organic honey

½ teaspoon ground cinnamon

⅛ teaspoon sea salt

3 bananas, peeled and cut into ¼-inch slices

1. Preheat the oven to 350°F.

2. Stir the coconut oil, lemon juice, honey, cinnamon, and salt in a medium bowl until well combined. Set aside.

3. Arrange the sliced bananas in an 8-by-8-inch baking dish.

4. Spoon the coconut oil mixture evenly over the bananas.

5. Bake the bananas until golden brown, about 20 minutes.

6. Let the bananas stand for 10 minutes to cool before serving.

DESSERTS

PER SERVING
CALORIES: 189
TOTAL FAT: 7 G
SODIUM: 61 MG
CARBS: 25 G
SUGAR: 14 G
PROTEIN: 1 G

MANGO GELATIN

MAKE AHEAD | KIDS' FAVORITE | QUICK+EASY

▶ Serves 4

▶ Prep time: 15 minutes, plus 2 hours to chill ▶ Cook time: 5 minutes

Mango is a luscious fruit with a sweet almost pine-like flavor and a vibrant sunny color. Mango is a rich source of vitamins A, C, and E as well as beta-carotene, amino acids, and iron. This nutrition profile means mangoes promote eye health and good digestion while reducing the risk of anemia and cancer. This charming gelled dessert can also be made with other thick fruit purées, such as strawberry or papaya.

4 teaspoons unflavored gelatin

1 cup water

1½ cups fresh mango purée

2 cups unsweetened organic coconut milk (for homemade, see page 258)

1. Add the gelatin and water to a small saucepan over medium heat and stir to combine.

2. Simmer the water until the gelatin dissolves, about 2 minutes. Do not boil. Remove the saucepan from the heat and set aside.

3. Whisk the mango purée and coconut milk in a small bowl until well combined.

4. Add the mango mixture to the gelatin mixture and whisk until well combined.

5. Pour the mango gelatin into 4 (6-ounce) ramekins and chill them in the refrigerator for 2 hours before serving.

6. Store the gelatin in a sealed container in the refrigerator for up to 2 days.

DESSERTS

PER SERVING
CALORIES: 100
TOTAL FAT: 2 G
SODIUM: 23 MG
CARBS: 14 G
SUGAR: 12 G
PROTEIN: 7 G

STEWED RHUBARB

MAKE AHEAD | GOOD FOR BATCHES

▶ Makes 7 cups (1 cup per serving)

▶ Prep time: 15 minutes ▶ Cook time: 1 hour

Fans of tart foods will love this easy dessert. You might want to have it for breakfast, and a snack, as well. Rhubarb is a vegetable often baked into pies and stewed like a fruit. Rhubarb is low in calories, high in vitamins A and K, and a good source of iron, calcium, and potassium. Rhubarb is usually available in early summer, and any extra stalks should be stored uncut in a sealed container in the refrigerator for up to 1 week. Never eat rhubarb leaves because they contain oxalic acid, which is toxic.

2 bunches rhubarb (about 10 cups), tops and bottoms removed

2 cups strawberries

½ cup water

2 tablespoons local organic honey

1 teaspoon ground cinnamon

1. Chop the rhubarb into 1-inch pieces.

2. Add the rhubarb, strawberries, water, honey, and cinnamon to a large stockpot over medium-high heat, and bring to a boil.

3. Reduce the heat to low and simmer until the rhubarb breaks down and the liquid reduces to a syrup, about 1 hour.

4. Serve the rhubarb warm.

5. Store any leftovers in a sealed container in the refrigerator for up to 1 week.

DESSERTS

PER SERVING

CALORIES: 120

TOTAL FAT: 0 G

SODIUM: 15 MG

CARBS: 29 G

SUGAR: 15 G

PROTEIN: 3 G

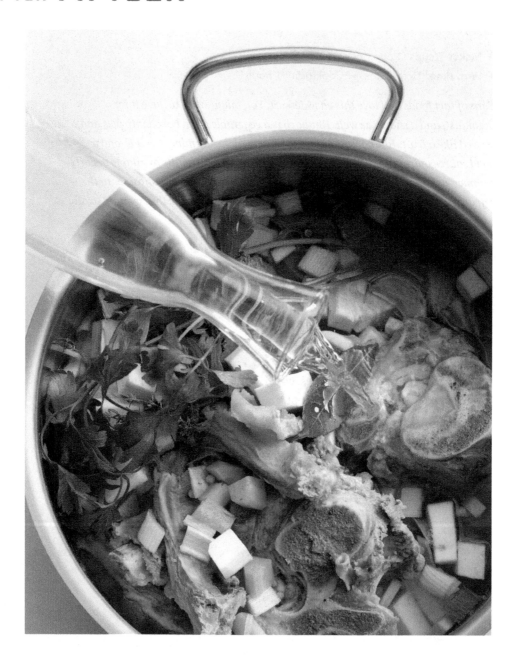

KITCHEN STAPLES

ROASTED BERRY JAM

FODMAP-FREE | MAKE AHEAD | KIDS' FAVORITE | QUICK+EASY | GOOD FOR BATCHES

- ▸ Makes 2 cups (2 tablespoons per serving)
- ▸ Prep time: 10 minutes, plus 8 hours to chill ▸ Cook time: 20 minutes

This jam has an intense berry taste that makes commercial jams seem dull in comparison. If you like a slightly sweeter jam or your berries are slightly under-ripe, you can stir in 1 tablespoon of maple syrup with the gelatin and zest. Strawberries are best in the spring, when they are in season, so find a local pick-your-own field and whip up a few batches of this delightful jam. Try to use your strawberries within two days of picking them, because a significant amount of vitamin C is lost after that time.

KITCHEN STAPLES

PER SERVING
CALORIES: 33
TOTAL FAT: 1 G
SODIUM: 4 MG
CARBS: 3 G
SUGAR: 1 G
PROTEIN: 2 G

½ pound whole strawberries, halved

½ pound fresh raspberries

2 tablespoons melted coconut oil

1 (2-teaspoon) package unflavored gelatin

2 teaspoons lemon zest

1. Preheat the oven to 350°F.

2. Line a baking sheet with parchment paper and set aside.

3. Toss the strawberries, raspberries, and coconut oil in a large bowl until well combined.

4. Transfer the berries to the baking sheet and spread them out in one layer.

5. Roast the berries for 15 minutes.

6. Spoon the berries back into the bowl and add the gelatin and lemon zest.

7. Mash the berries up until they are the desired consistency and the other ingredients are well combined.

8. Spoon the jam into containers and place the containers in the refrigerator for at least 8 hours.

9. Store the jam in a sealed container in the refrigerator for up to 2 weeks.

COCONUT BUTTER

FODMAP-FREE | MAKE AHEAD | KIDS' FAVORITE | QUICK+EASY | GOOD FOR BATCHES

- ▸ Makes 2 cups (1 tablespoon per serving)
- ▸ Prep time: 20 minutes

You might be wondering what the difference is between coconut butter and coconut oil. Coconut oil is extracted from the meat of the coconut and coconut butter is the meat that has been processed until it is buttery, like any other nut butter, such as peanut butter. You can spread coconut butter on fresh fruit or celery stalks, top other foods with it, and add it to smoothies and dressings for a creamy coconut accent. You really can't get the right creamy texture without a food processor or a blender, so if you don't have either one, look for commercially prepared coconut butter in the organic section of the grocery store.

6 cups shredded unsweetened coconut

1. Place the coconut in a food processor or a blender and process on high speed until the coconut becomes very thick and buttery, scraping down the sides, about 15 minutes. Give your machine a rest every few minutes.

2. Store the coconut butter in a sealed glass jar in a cool, dark place for up to 2 months.

KITCHEN STAPLES

PER SERVING
CALORIES: 150
TOTAL FAT: 13 G
SODIUM: 8 MG
CARBS: 7 G
SUGAR: 1 G
PROTEIN: 2 G

HOMEMADE COCONUT MILK

▸ Makes 4 cups (½ cup per serving)
▸ Prep time: 15 minutes ▸ Cook time: 5 minutes

You may never buy commercially prepared coconut milk again after making this simple recipe. This milk tastes better than the commercial kind and is economical, and you will have lots of coconut pulp leftover to make into coconut flour. Coconut milk has antibacterial, antiviral, and antifungal properties that help support a healthy immune system.

4 cups filtered water
2 cups shredded unsweetened coconut

**KITCHEN
STAPLES**

PER SERVING
CALORIES: 23
TOTAL FAT: 2 G
SODIUM: 8 MG
CARBS: 1 G
SUGAR: 1 G
PROTEIN: 0 G

1. Place the water in a large saucepan over medium-high heat.

2. Heat the water until it is very hot but not scalding, about 5 minutes.

3. Add the coconut and hot water to a blender and process on high until the mixture is creamy, about 4 minutes.

4. Pour the liquid through a fine mesh sieve to remove the majority of the shredded coconut.

5. Pour the strained liquid through a double layer of fine cheesecloth to catch the remaining coconut. Squeeze the solid bits in the cloth to get all the liquid.

6. Store the coconut milk in a sealed container in the refrigerator for 3 to 4 days.

7. Shake the coconut milk before each use.

HOMEMADE COCONUT YOGURT

FODMAP-FREE | MAKE AHEAD | KIDS' FAVORITE

- ▸ Makes 4 cups (½ cup per serving)
- ▸ Prep time: 30 minutes, plus 12 hours to ferment

Yogurt is very simple to make, but you do need a catalyst to start the fermentation process. If you want to make your own yogurt completely from scratch, you can grow the kefir grains for the coconut kefir. You can buy kefir grains online from several companies. Simply follow the directions to grow your own grains, and experiment until you have the finished product you want. Store-bought coconut kefir works, too, so look for that product in the organic section of your grocery store for a quicker yogurt process.

16 ounces shredded unsweetened coconut

¼ cup coconut kefir

¼ cup coconut water

¼ cup freshly squeezed lemon juice

1. Place the coconut, coconut kefir, coconut water, and lemon juice in a blender and process until smooth and creamy.

2. Transfer the mixture to a jar or glass bowl and cover it with a fine-mesh cheesecloth.

3. Leave the yogurt mixture out at room temperature for 12 hours.

4. Stir the yogurt, seal the container, and store it in the refrigerator for up to 1 week.

KITCHEN STAPLES

PER SERVING

CALORIES: 207

TOTAL FAT: 19 G

SODIUM: 14 MG

CARBS: 9 G

SUGAR: 4 G

PROTEIN: 2 G

EASY GUACAMOLE

MAKE AHEAD | KIDS' FAVORITE | QUICK+EASY

▸ Serves 8
▸ Prep time: 15 minutes

Avocados are the fruit of an evergreen tree. They're high in vitamin K, fiber, and carotenoids that can be turned into vitamin A in the body. The highest concentration of carotenoids is found in the darker green flesh of the avocado, right below the skin, so peel your fruit carefully to preserve this layer. This dip is lovely with cut-up vegetables, or use it to top soups, stews, and casseroles.

3 avocados, halved, peeled, and pitted
¼ sweet onion, finely chopped
2 tablespoons freshly squeezed lime juice
1 teaspoon minced fresh garlic
¼ cup chopped fresh cilantro
Pinch sea salt

1. Place the avocado halves in a medium bowl and mash them coarsely with a potato masher.

2. Add the onion, lime juice, garlic, cilantro, and salt, and stir until well combined.

3. Store the guacamole in a sealed container in the refrigerator for up to 3 days.

KITCHEN STAPLES

PER SERVING
CALORIES: 158
TOTAL FAT: 15 G
SODIUM: 36 MG
CARBS: 8 G
SUGAR: 1 G
PROTEIN: 1 G

HERB-SPINACH PESTO

MAKE AHEAD | QUICK+EASY | **GOOD FOR BATCHES**

▶ Makes 1½ cups (2 tablespoons per serving)

▶ Prep time: 15 minutes

Pesto can be stirred into soups, used as a marinade for meats, fish, or poultry, or tossed with vegetable "noodles." Most commercially prepared pesto is a blend of herbs, garlic, nuts, and olive oil. This recipe has spinach as a base, which adds vitamins A and K, iron, protein, and fiber to the pesto. Spinach supports the immune and nervous systems and may help reduce the risk of cardiovascular disease. Nutritional yeast is a cheesy tasting, deactivated yeast organism that does not grow or froth like the yeast you use for bread. It can be found in most grocery stores in the organic section or at a health food store.

1 cup packed spinach

1 cup packed fresh basil leaves

2 garlic cloves

2 teaspoons nutritional yeast

¼ cup extra-virgin olive oil

2 tablespoons water (optional)

1. Place the spinach, basil, garlic, and nutritional yeast in a food processor and pulse until the mixture is finely chopped, about 3 minutes. If you don't have a food processor, you can use an old-fashioned mortar and pestle to crush everything perfectly.

2. With the food processor running, drizzle the olive oil into the pesto until a thick paste forms, scraping down the sides at least once.

3. Add the water if the pesto is too thick.

4. Store the pesto in a sealed container in the refrigerator for up to 1 week.

KITCHEN STAPLES

PER SERVING

CALORIES: 40

TOTAL FAT: 4 G

SODIUM: 3 MG

CARBS: 1 G

SUGAR: 0 G

PROTEIN: 1 G

NATURALLY FERMENTED PICKLES

MAKE AHEAD | KIDS' FAVORITE | QUICK+EASY | GOOD FOR BATCHES

▸ Makes 2 quarts (2 pickles per serving)
▸ Prep time: 15 minutes, plus 2 weeks to ferment ▸ Cook time: 15 minutes

The small cucumbers used for pickles are not baby cucumbers but a variety that is fully mature when it is about four to five inches long. These are called pickling cucumbers, or kirbys. The most important part of pickling is to be sure everything you use is scrupulously clean. This includes your own hands, the jars and lids, and the pot you boil the water and salt in for the brine. The cucumbers should also be blemish-free, with no soft or discolored spots, to create safe and deliciously crisp pickles.

KITCHEN STAPLES

PER SERVING
CALORIES: 81
TOTAL FAT: 1 G
SODIUM: 947 MG
CARBS: 19 G
SUGAR: 0 G
PROTEIN: 3 G

20 to 24 (4-inch) pickling cucumbers
4 garlic cloves, smashed
4 bay leaves
3 cups filtered water, plus more as needed
¼ cup sea salt

1. Sterilize two 1-quart mason jars and their lids by dipping them in boiling water using tongs. Carefully set aside. Thoroughly wash everything you will be using.

2. Pack the jars halfway full with the cucumbers, then add 1 garlic clove and 1 bay leaf to each jar. Press down firmly.

3. Pack the remaining cucumbers in the jars and add 1 garlic clove and 1 bay leaf to the top of each jar. Leave about 2 inches of free space at the top of each jar. Set aside.

4. Pour the filtered water and the salt into a saucepan set over medium heat.

5. Stir until the salt is dissolved, then remove the pan from the heat.

6. Pour 1½ cups of the brine into each jar.

7. Fill the jars with additional filtered water, if needed, so that the contents are covered by about 1 inch of water. Seal the jars.

8. Shake the jars and place them in a cool, dark place for 2 weeks. Check the jars once a day to see if pressure is building up. If the center of the lid can't be pressed down, open the jar by unscrewing the lid. This is called burping, and it allows the built-up gasses to escape.

9. After 2 weeks, store the fermented pickles in the sealed containers in the refrigerator for up to 2 months.

NATURALLY FERMENTED SAUERKRAUT

- ▸ Makes 2 quarts (½ cup per serving)
- ▸ Prep time: 45 minutes, plus 5 to 10 days to ferment

The heat-free fermentation method used to make this tangy vegetables staple is called lacto-fermentation. This process has been used for centuries to preserve food and requires only vegetables such as cabbage, plus salt and water. Fermentation produces beneficial probiotic bacteria that assist in the digestive process and promote gut health.

2 heads green cabbage, finely shredded (set aside about 8 large outer leaves)
¼ cup sea salt

KITCHEN STAPLES

PER SERVING
CALORIES: 45
TOTAL FAT: 0 G
SODIUM: 1,436 MG
CARBS: 10 G
SUGAR: 6 G
PROTEIN: 2 G

1. Sterilize three or four 1-quart mason jars and their lids by dipping them in boiling water using tongs. Carefully set aside. Thoroughly wash everything you will be using.

2. Place the shredded cabbage in a very large bowl, layering it with the salt.

3. Massage and scrunch the cabbage with your hands until liquid starts to purge out, and the cabbage becomes limp and watery, about 10 minutes.

4. Pack the cabbage into the clean jars and pour any leftover liquid in the bowl into the jars.

5. Cover the cabbage in the jars with the reserved leaves so that the shredded vegetable stays submerged in the liquid.

6. Place a small jelly jar filled with clean rocks or marbles on the leaves in the tops of the mason jars to weigh down the sauerkraut.

7. Cover the mouth of each jar with a square of fine mesh cheesecloth secured with a rubber band (leave off the jar lids). Place the jars in a cool, dark place.

8. For the first 24 hours, press down every few hours on the jelly jars to release more liquid.

9. After 24 hours there should be enough liquid to cover the sauerkraut, so you don't need to press it down any longer.

10. Ferment the sauerkraut for between 5 and 10 days, depending on how tangy you want your finished product.

11. When your sauerkraut has the perfect taste, remove the weighted jars, add the clean lids, and store the jars in the refrigerator for up to 3 months.

CHICKEN BONE BROTH

MAKE AHEAD | GOOD FOR BATCHES

▸ Makes 8 to 10 cups (1 cup per serving)

▸ Prep time: 15 minutes ▸ Cook time: 28 to 36 hours

This recipe makes a great deal of broth, so if you don't need quite so much, scale the recipe down. The apple cider vinegar might seem like a strange addition, but it helps draw the nutrients out of the bones, so don't omit this ingredient. The quantity and variety of vegetables used in this broth adds flavor and some nutrients, but if you want a plain chicken broth, use just the carcasses, vinegar, and water.

PER SERVING
CALORIES: 30
TOTAL FAT: 3 G
SODIUM: 90 MG
CARBS: 0 G
SUGAR: 1 G
PROTEIN: 1 G

2 or 3 chicken carcasses

2 tablespoons apple cider vinegar

1 gallon cold water

3 carrots, peeled and roughly chopped

3 celery stalks, cut into quarters

1 sweet onion, peeled and quartered

4 garlic cloves, smashed

1. Preheat the oven to 350°F.

2. Place the chicken carcasses in a deep baking pan and roast them in the oven for 30 minutes.

3. Transfer the roasted carcasses to a large stockpot and add the vinegar and water.

4. Let the mixture stand for 30 minutes.

5. Place the pot on high heat and bring to a boil.

6. Reduce the heat to low and gently simmer the chicken bone broth, stirring every few hours, for 24 hours.

7. Add the carrots, celery, onion, and garlic, and bring to a boil again.

8. Reduce the heat and simmer the broth for 8 more hours, stirring several times.

9. Remove the pot from the heat and cool slightly.

10. Remove any large bones with tongs, then strain the broth through a fine-mesh sieve and discard the solid bits.

11. Pour the broth into jars and allow it to cool completely.

12. Store the broth in sealed jars in the refrigerator for up to 5 days or in the freezer for up to 3 months.

EASY BEEF BONE BROTH

▸ Makes 8 to 10 cups (1 cup per serving)

▸ Prep time: 15 minutes ▸ Cook time: 48 hours

This broth is not just a staple; it is an essential for the Autoimmune Paleo Diet. Bone broth is rich in gelatin, which is helps heal the gut, as well as collagen and amino acids, which promote healthy joints and ligaments. The minerals in bone broth are easily accessible to the body and include calcium, magnesium, and phosphorus; it also contains glucosamine, a component of connective tissue. Beef bones should not be expensive, and you can usually buy bones of pasture-raised animals from reputable butchers and farmers' markets. Use the bone broth in your recipes and as a healthy drink in the mornings or whenever you need a boost.

KITCHEN STAPLES

PER SERVING
CALORIES: 80
TOTAL FAT: 5 G
SODIUM: 40 MG
CARBS: 0 G
SUGAR: 0 G
PROTEIN: 4 G

2 to 3 pounds beef bones (beef marrow, knuckle bones, ribs, and any other bones)

1 sweet onion, peeled and quartered

2 carrots, peeled and roughly chopped

2 tablespoons apple cider vinegar

1 gallon water

1. Preheat the oven to 350°F.

2. Place the bones in a deep baking pan and roast them in the oven for 30 minutes.

3. Transfer the roasted bones to a large stockpot and add the onion, carrots, vinegar, and water, making sure the bones are covered.

4. Let the mixture stand for 30 minutes.

5. Place the pot on high heat and bring to a boil.

6. Reduce the heat to low and simmer the bone broth for 48 hours. Check the broth every half hour, at least for the first few hours, for impurities floating on the top of the liquid. Skim the impurities off the top with a spoon.

7. Remove the pot from the heat and cool slightly.

8. Remove any large bones with tongs, then strain the broth through a fine-mesh sieve and discard the solid bits.

9. Pour the broth into jars and allow it to cool completely.

10. Store the broth in sealed jars in the refrigerator for up to 5 days, or in the freezer for up to 3 months.

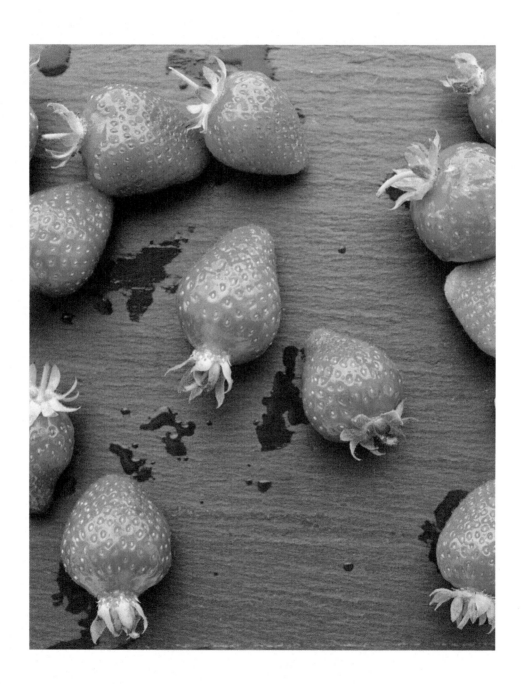

GLOSSARY

amino acids: The building blocks of protein. Your body breaks protein down into amino acids in order to use them.

antibody: Also called an immunoglobulin. A specialized protein produced by a B cell in response to an antigen. The antibody binds to the antigen, marking it for destruction.

antigen: A foreign body, such as bacteria, cancer cells, viruses, or toxins, that is marked by the immune system for destruction.

anti-inflammatory: A property of a substance or treatment that counteracts or reduces inflammation.

antinutrient: A compound or substance that interferes with the absorption of nutrients.

antioxidants: Nutrients found in vegetables, fruits, oils, and algae that protect the body from free radicals, which may cause cell damage; free radicals have been linked to cancer, diabetes, and other diseases.

autoantibody: An antibody that attacks the body's own organs, tissues, and cells.

autoimmune disease: A condition in which the immune system, which protects the body from bacteria, viruses, and other outside invaders, attacks the body itself instead.

autoimmunity: An immune response against the body's own cells and tissues.

B cell: An immune cell that is a type of lymphocyte and produces antibodies that bind to antigens.

calorie: The unit of measurement of the energy in food. Higher calories mean more energy; if you eat more energy than you use, your body stores it as fat. A calorie from fat contains the same amount of energy as a calorie from carbohydrates.

carbohydrates (carbs): One of the main food energy sources used by your body. Carbohydrates are either simple or complex. Simple carbs are broken down by the body quickly and can cause blood sugar fluctuations. They have less nutritional value and include white sugar, honey, and white flour. Complex carbs take longer to digest and are full of fiber, minerals, and vitamins. Healthy complex carb sources include vegetables and fruit.

circadian rhythm: Biological functions that follow a 24-hour clock, such as tissue repair, digestion, and growth. Cells in the brain control the rhythm and hormones that circulate through the body, synchronizing the individual cells' 24-hour clocks with the brain.

cortisol: The main stress hormone, produced in the adrenal cortex. It also helps regulate the immune system and metabolism.

cytokines: Chemical substances that can act as messengers to turn inflammation on or off in the body.

enterocyte: Also called intestinal absorptive cells. Specialized epithelial barrier cells in the gut that transport nutrients from the gut to the body.

essential amino acids: The amino acids that your body can't produce itself or not in the quantities it needs. There are nine essential amino acids, which must come from food or supplements.

essential fatty acids: Fats that the body can't produce itself. These are essential to the workings in the body and must be obtained from food. Omega-3 fatty acids and omega-6 fatty acids are the most commonly known.

flare-up: The serious, sudden onset of autoimmune disease symptoms or a worsening of existing symptoms.

FODMAPs: A group of carbohydrates that some people cannot digest easily, which means the carbs are not absorbed completely in the small intestine. FODMAPs (fermentable oligosaccharides, disaccharides, monosaccharides, and polyols) move through the digestive tract into the large intestine, where they ferment when digested by the gut microflora. This fermentation creates bloating, gas, cramps, pain, diarrhea, and constipation for people who are sensitive to these foods.

free radicals: Oxygen or nitrogen molecules that do not have electrons in complete sets. They cause damage in the body because they take electrons from surrounding cells to complete the electron set. Too many free radicals can contribute to the development of heart disease, dementia, cancer, and diabetes.

gliadin: A protein of gluten found in cereal grains such as wheat.

gluten: A protein found mostly in cereal grains. Many people are sensitive to gluten and must avoid all foods containing it.

glycemic index: A measure of how fast your blood sugar levels rise after eating a particular food.

glycemic load: A measurement that indicates the carbohydrate content of a food based on its glycemic index.

grass-fed meat: Meat produced from animals that are raised in pastures and allowed to graze naturally.

hormones: Chemical messengers excreted into the blood, which carries them to organs and tissues. There, they regulate a wide variety of physical processes, including growth, metabolism, sexual function, and mood.

immune system: The system that defends the body against attacks from foreign invaders such as bacteria, viruses, and other pathogens.

immunosuppressive drugs: Drugs that are used to treat autoimmune diseases by suppressing the immune system.

intestinal permeability: Also called leaky gut. When the wall of the gut is permeable because the enterocytes (cells that line the gut) or the bonds between the enterocytes have tiny holes that allow the contents of the gut to leak through into the body. This leakage can include pathogens, incomplete proteins, waste products, and friendly bacteria.

lectin: Carbohydrate-binding proteins found in plants and animals.

leukocyte: A type of white blood cell.

lymphocyte: A type of white blood cell that includes B cells and T cells.

macronutrients: The categories of nutrients your body uses for essential tasks. They include protein, carbohydrates, and fat and make up the main part of your diet.

micronutrients: Nutrients, such as vitamins and minerals, that your body needs in small quantities.

monocyte: A type of white blood cell.

natural killer cell: A type of white blood cell that responds quickly to specifically attack virally infected cells.

nonsteroidal anti-inflammatory drugs (NSAIDs): Drugs used to reduce inflammation and pain associated with joints.

omega-3 fatty acids: A group of three fats (ALA, EPA, and DHA) that are essential for good health and aren't synthesized by your body. They help cell walls form and assist with almost every cell activity. They are found mostly in fatty fish.

omega-6 fatty acids: Unsaturated fatty acids, such as linoleic and arachidonic acid, that aren't synthesized by your body but are essential to your health because they can help fight cancer and diseases like arthritis.

omega ratio: The ratio of omega-3 fatty acids to omega-6 fatty acids in food. Ideally, the amount of omega-3 should be higher than or equal to the amount of omega-6. In the modern Western diet, most people get too much omega-6 fatty acids and not enough omega-3 fatty acids. This dietary imbalance may explain the rise of diseases that stem from inflammation in the body, such as asthma, coronary heart disease, many forms of cancer, autoimmunity, and neurodegenerative diseases. The imbalance between omega-3 and omega-6 fatty acids may also contribute to obesity and even depression.

pathogen: Something that can make you sick, such as a virus, parasite, or bacteria.

phytonutrients: Chemical compounds found only in plants that have many beneficial effects, including cutting the risk of diseases such as cancer, cardiovascular disease, and stroke.

probiotics: Live bacteria that aid in digestion and help eliminate unhealthy bacteria in your body.

pro-inflammatory: Something that causes inflammation.

protease: An enzyme that breaks proteins apart.

protease inhibitor: A substance that blocks the breakdown of protein.

protein: An essential nutrient that your body uses for many functions, including maintaining and building lean muscle mass.

pseudograin: The edible seeds of broadleaf plants; they resemble grains but are not in the same biological group.

saponin: A substance in some plants that has detergent-like qualities.

T cell: A type of lymphocyte (white blood cell) that identifies, attacks, and destroys foreign agents in the body.

APPENDIX ONE
TRACK YOUR REACTIONS

When trying to pinpoint trigger foods in your diet, it is important to keep a log of everything you eat and any reactions you have to the food. This should ideally be done before you start the diet, to get an informed idea of what might be problem foods for you. You should also track the elimination phase, especially if you are prone to cheating a little. The log is meant to track both positive and negative reactions such as a symptom clearing up or worsening. Log the foods you've eaten, the time of day, any symptoms you experience, and when.

Weekly Food Diary

		DAY 1	DAY 2	DAY 3	DAY 4	DAY 5	DAY 6	DAY 7
MORNING	Foods							
	Symptoms							
AFTERNOON	Foods							
	Symptoms							
EVENING	Foods							
	Symptoms							

APPENDIX TWO
THE DIRTY DOZEN AND THE CLEAN FIFTEEN

A nonprofit and environmental watchdog organization called Environmental Working Group (EWG) looks at data supplied by the US Department of Agriculture (USDA) and the Food and Drug Administration (FDA) about pesticide residues and compiles a list each year of the best and worst pesticide loads found in commercial crops. You can use these lists to decide which fruits and vegetables to buy organic to minimize your exposure to pesticides and which produce is considered safe enough to skip the organics. This does not mean they are pesticide-free, though, so wash these fruits and vegetables thoroughly.

These lists change every year, so make sure you look up the most recent before you fill your shopping cart. You'll find the most recent lists as well as a guide to pesticides in produce at EWG.org/FoodNews.

2014 Dirty Dozen

Apples	Peaches	*In addition to the dirty dozen, the EWG added two produce contaminated with highly toxic organophosphate insecticides:*
Celery	Potatoes	
Cherry tomatoes	Snap peas (imported)	
Cucumbers	Spinach	
Grapes	Strawberries	Blueberries (domestic)
Nectarines (imported)	Sweet bell peppers	Hot peppers

2014 Clean Fifteen

Asparagus	Eggplants	Papayas
Avocados	Grapefruits	Pineapples
Cabbage	Kiwis	Sweet corn
Cantaloupes (domestic)	Mangoes	Sweet peas (frozen)
Cauliflower	Onions	Sweet potatoes

CONVERSION TABLES

Volume Equivalents (Liquid)

U.S. STANDARD	U.S. STANDARD (OUNCES)	METRIC (APPROXIMATE)
2 tablespoons	1 fl. oz.	30 mL
¼ cup	2 fl. oz.	60 mL
½ cup	4 fl. oz.	120 mL
1 cup	8 fl. oz.	240 mL
1½ cups	12 fl. oz.	355 mL
2 cups or 1 pint	16 fl. oz.	475 mL
4 cups or 1 quart	32 fl. oz.	1 L
1 gallon	128 fl. oz.	4 L

Oven Temperatures

FAHRENHEIT (F)	CELSIUS (C) (APPROXIMATE)
250	120
300	150
325	165
350	180
375	190
400	200
425	220
450	230

Volume Equivalents (Dry)

U.S. STANDARD	METRIC (APPROXIMATE)
⅛ teaspoon	0.5 mL
¼ teaspoon	1 mL
½ teaspoon	2 mL
¾ teaspoon	4 mL
1 teaspoon	5 mL
1 tablespoon	15 mL
¼ cup	59 mL
⅓ cup	79 mL
½ cup	118 mL
⅔ cup	156 mL
¾ cup	177 mL
1 cup	235 mL
2 cups or 1 pint	475 mL
3 cups	700 mL
4 cups or 1 quart	1 L
½ gallon	2 L
1 gallon	4 L

Weight Equivalents

U.S. STANDARD	METRIC (APPROXIMATE)
½ ounce	15 g
1 ounce	30 g
2 ounces	60 g
4 ounces	115 g
8 ounces	225 g
12 ounces	340 g
16 ounces or 1 pound	455 g

REFERENCES

Abbas, Abul K., Andrew H. Lichtman, and Shiv Pillai. *Basic Immunology: Functions and Disorders of the Immune System*. 4th ed. Philadelphia: Saunders, 2012.

American Autoimmune Related Diseases Association. "Autoimmune Statistics." Accessed June 15, 2014. http://www.aarda.org/autoimmune-information/autoimmune-statistics/.

Assimakopoulos, Stelios F., Ismini Papageorgiou, and Aristidis Charonis. "Enterocytes' Tight Junctions: From Molecules to Diseases." *World Journal of Gastrointestinal Pathophysiology* 2, no. 6 (December 2011): 123–37. doi:10.4291/wjgp.v2.i6.123.

Baatar, Dolgor, Kalpesh Patel, and Dennis D. Taub. "The Effects of Ghrelin on Inflammation and the Immune System." *Molecular and Cellular Endocrinology* 340, no. 1 (June 2011): 44–58. doi:10.1016/j.mce.2011.04.019.

Bahna, Sami L. "Food Challenge Procedure: Optimal Choices for Clinical Practice." *Allergy and Asthma Proceedings* 28, no. 6 (November–December 2007): 640–46. doi:10.2500/aap.2007.28.3068.

Ballantyne, Sarah. *The Paleo Approach: Reverse Autoimmune Disease and Heal Your Body*. Las Vegas: Victory Belt Publishing, 2013.

Bennett, M. P., J. M. Zeller, L. Rosenberg, and J. McCann. "The Effect of Mirthful Laughter on Stress and Natural Killer Cell Activity." *Alternative Therapies in Health and Medicine* 9, no. 2 (March-April 2003): 38–45. http://www.ncbi.nlm.nih.gov/pubmed/12652882.

Biesiekierski, Jessica R., Evan D. Newnham, Peter M. Irving, Jacqueline S. Barrett, Melissa Haines, James D. Doecke, Susan J. Shepherd, Jane G. Muir, and Peter R. Gibson. "Gluten Causes Gastrointestinal Symptoms in Subjects without Celiac Disease: A Double-Blind Randomized Placebo-Controlled Trial." *American Journal of Gastroenterology* 106, no. 3 (March 2011): 508–14. doi:10.1038/ajg.2010.487.

Bisht, Babita, Warren G. Darling, Ruth E. Grossmann, E. Torage Shivapour, Susan K. Lutgendorf, Linda G. Snetselaar, Michael J. Hall, M. Bridget Zimmerman, and Terry L. Wahls. "A Multimodal Intervention for Patients with Secondary Progressive Multiple Sclerosis: Feasibility and Effect on Fatigue." *Journal of Alternative and Complementary Medicine* 20, no. 5 (May 2014): 347–55. doi:10.1089/acm.2013.0188.

Bjarnason, I. "Intestinal Permeability." *Gut* 35 (1994): S18–S22. http://gut.bmj.com/content/35/1_Suppl/S18.full.pdf+html?sid=f63dea71-ec5d-4813-b139-609cbbf148c0.

Brown, Jonathon D., and Judith M. Siegel. "Exercise as a Buffer of Life Stress: A Prospective Study of Adolescent Health." *Health Psychology* 7, no. 4 (1988): 341–53. doi:10.1037/0278-6133.7.4.341.

Brunstrom, J. M., and G. L. Mitchell. "Effects of Distraction on the Development of Satiety." *British Journal of Nutrition* 96, no. 4 (October

2006): 761–9. http://www.ncbi.nlm.nih.gov/pubmed/17010237.

Bures, Jan, Jiri Cyrany, Darina Kohoutova, Miroslav Förstl, Stanislav Rejchrt, Jaroslav Kvetina, Viktor Vorisek, and Marcela Kopacova. "Small Intestinal Bacterial Overgrowth Syndrome." *World Journal of Gatroenterology* 16, no. 24 (June 2010): 2978–90. http://www.ncbi.nlm.nih.gov/pmc/articles/PMC2890937.

Chighizola, Cecilia, and Pier Luigi Meroni. "The Role of Environmental Estrogens and Autoimmunity." *Autoimmunity Reviews* 11, nos. 6–7 (May 2002): 493–501. doi:10.1016/j.autrev.2011.11.027.

Coelho, Justina. "Ten Famous People on the Paleo Diet." *LA Weekly*. January 16, 2014. http://www.laweekly.com/squidink/2014/01/16/ten-famous-people-on-the-paleo-diet?showFullText=true.

Cordain, Loren. "Cereal Grains: Humanity's Double-Edged Sword." *World Review of Nutrition and Dietetics* 84 (1999): 19–73. doi:10.1159/000059677.

———. "The Nutritional Characteristics of a Contemporary Diet Based upon Paleolithic Food Groups." *Journal of American Nutraceutical Association* 5, no. 3 (Summer 2002): 15–24. http://www.docstoc.com/docs/157671539/The-Nutritional-Characteristics-of-a-Contemporary-Diet-Based-Upon-Paleolithic-Food-Groupsabstract4.

Cutolo, M., B. Seriolo, C. Craviotto, C. Pizzorni, and A. Sulli. "Circadian Rhythms in RA." *Annals of the Rheumatic Diseases* 62 (2003): 593–96. doi:10.1136/ard.62.7.593.

Cutolo, Maurizio. "Vitamin D or Hormone D Deficiency in Autoimmune Rheumatic Diseases, Including Undifferentiated Connective Tissue Disease." *Arthritis Research and Therapy* 10 (2008). doi:10.1186/ar2552.

Environmental Working Group (EWG). "All 48 Fruits and Vegetables with Pesticide Residue Data." April 2014. http://www.ewg.org/foodnews/list.php.

———. "EWG's 2014 Shopper's Guide to Pesticides in Produce." April 2014. http://www.ewg.org/foodnews/.

Fasano, Alessio. "Leaky Gut and Autoimmune Diseases." *Clinical Reviews in Allergy and Immunology* 42, no. 1 (February 2012): 71–8. doi:10.1007/s12016-011-8291-x.

Flanigan, Jessica. AIP Lifestyle website. Accessed July 18, 2014. http://aiplifestyle.com.

Francis, George, Zohar Kerem, Harinder P. S. Makkar, and Klaus Becker. "The Biological Action of Saponins in Animal Systems: A Review." *British Journal of Nutrition* 88, no. 6 (December 2002): 587–605. doi:10.1079/BJN2002725.

Frey, Danielle J., Monika Fleshner, and Kenneth P. Wright Jr. "The Effects of 40 Hours of Total Sleep Deprivation on Inflammatory Markers in Healthy Young Adults." *Brain, Behavior, and Immunity* 21, no. 8 (November 2007): 1050–7. doi:10.1016/j.bbi.2007.04.003.

Gibson, Peter R., and Susan J. Shepherd. "Food Choice as a Key Management Strategy for Functional Gastrointestinal Symptoms." *American Journal of Gastroenterology* 107 (May 2012): 657–66. doi:10.1038/ajg.2012.49.

Gupta, Y. P. "Anti-Nutritional and Toxic Factors in Food Legumes: A Review." *Plant Foods for Human Nutrition* 37, no. 3 (1987): 201–28. doi:10.1007/BF01091786.

Haas, E. M., and B. Levin. *Staying Healthy with Nutrition. The Complete Guide to Diet and Nutritional Medicine.* Berkeley, CA: Celestial Arts, 2006.

Halmos, Emma P., Victoria A. Power, Susan J. Shepherd, Peter R. Gibson, and Jane G. Muir. "A Diet Low in FODMAPs Reduces Symptoms of Irritable Bowel Syndrome." *Gastroenterology* 146, no. 1 (January 2014): 67–75. doi:10.1053/j.gastro.2013.09.046.

Holick, M. F. "Sunlight and Vitamin D for Bone Health and Prevention of Autoimmune Diseases, Cancers, and Cardiovascular Disease." *American Journal of Clinical Nutrition* 80, no. 6 (December 2004): 1678S–88S. http://ajcn.nutrition.org/content/80/6/1678S.long.

Holt-Lunstad, J., W. A. Birmingham, and K. C. Light. "Influence of a 'Warm Touch' Support Enhancement Intervention among Married Couples on Ambulatory Blood Pressure, Oxytocin, Alpha Amylase, and Cortisol." *Psychosomatic Medicine* 70, no. 9 (November 2008): 976–85. http://www.ncbi.nlm.nih.gov/pubmed/18842740.

Jirillo, Emilio, Felicita Jirillo, and Thea Magrone. "Healthy Effects Exerted by Prebiotics, Probiotics, and Symbiotics with Special Reference to Their Impact on the Immune System." *International Journal for Vitamin and Nutrition Research* 82, no. 3 (June 2012): 200–8. doi:10.1024/0300-9831/a000112.

Klaus, Jochen, Ulrike Spaniol, Guido Adler, Richard A. Mason, Max Reinshagen, and Christian von Tirpitz. "Small Intestinal Bacterial Overgrowth Mimicking Acute Flare as a Pitfall in Patients with Crohn's Disease." *BMC Gastroenterology* 9 (July 2009). doi:10.1186/1471-230X-9-61.

Levinson, Warren. *Review of Medical Microbiology and Immunology.* 12th ed. New York: McGraw-Hill Medical, 2012.

Machello, Martin J. "Palatability and Nutrient Composition of Grass-Finished Bison." Bison Producers of Alberta. Accessed June 17, 2014. http://bisoncentre.com/index.php/producers-2/resource-library/ibc2000-proceedings/bison-meat-information/-palatability-and-nutrient-composition-of-grass-finished-bison.

Mastorakos, George, Maria Pavlatou, Evanthia Diamanti-Kandarakis, and George P. Chrousos. "Exercise and the Stress System." *Hormones* 4, no. 2 (2005): 73–89. http://www.hormones.gr/57/article/article.html.

Merkes, Monika. "Mindfulness-Based Stress Reduction for People with Chronic Diseases." *Australian Journal of Primary Health* 16, no. 3 (2010): 200–10. doi:10.1071/PY09063.

Miles, M. P., W. J. Kraemer, B. C. Nindl, D. S. Grove, S. K. Leach, K. Dohi, J. O. Marx, J. S. Volek, and A. M. Mastro. "Strength, Workload, Anaerobic Intensity and the Immune Response to Resistance Exercise in Women." *Acta Physiologica Scandinavica* 178, no. 2 (June 2003): 155–63. doi:10.1046/j.1365-201X.2003.01124.x.

Moore, Elaine A. *Autoimmune Diseases and Their Environmental Triggers.* Jefferson, NC: McFarland & Company, 2002.

Palmer, Sharon. "Is There a Link between Nutrition and Autoimmune Disease?" *Today's Dietitian* 13, no 11 (November 2011): 36. http://www.todaysdietitian.com/newarchives/110211p36.shtml.

Scarlata, Kate. "Small Intestinal Bacterial Overgrowth—What to Do When Unwelcome

Microbes Invade." *Today's Dietitian* 13, no. 4 (April 2011): 46. http://www.todaysdietitian.com/newarchives/040511p46.shtml.

Sekirov, Inna, Shannon L. Russell, L. Caetano M. Antunes, and B. Brett Finlay. "Gut Microbiota in Health and Disease." *Physiological Reviews* 90 (July 2010): 859–904. doi:10.1152/physrev.00045.2009.

Shepherd, Susan J., Francis C. Parker, Jane G. Muir, and Peter R. Gibson. "Dietary Triggers of Abdominal Symptoms in Patients with Irritable Bowel Syndrome: Randomized Placebo-Controlled Evidence." *Clinical Gastroenterology and Hepatology* 6, no. 7 (July 2008): 765–71. doi:10.1016/j.cgh.2008.02.058.

Shiau, S. Y., and G. W. Chang. "Effects of Dietary Fiber on Fecal Mucinase and Beta-glucuronidase Activity in Rats." *Journal of Nutrition* 113, no. 1 (January 1983): 138–44.

http://www.ncbi.nlm.nih.gov/pubmed/6296339.

Sterczala, Adam J. "The Stress Response to an Acute Heavy Resistance Exercise Protocol." Master's thesis. University of Connecticut, 2014. http://digitalcommons.uconn.edu/cgi/viewcontent.cgi?article=1660&context=gs_theses.

US Food and Drug Administration (FDA). 2009 Summary Report on Antimicrobials Sold or Distributed for Use in Food-Producing Animals. Silver Spring, ID: US Food and Drug Administration, 2009.

Whelan, K., and E. M. Quigley. "Probiotics in the Management of Irritable Bowel Syndrome and Inflammatory Bowel Disease." *Current Opinion in Gastroenterology* 29, no. 2 (March 2013): 184–9. doi:10.1097/MOG.0b013e32835d7bba.

RECIPE INDEX

INDEX

Z

CPSIA information can be obtained
at www.ICGtesting.com
Printed in the USA
LVOW05s1614060118
562079LV00001B/1/P